Glossary of abbreviations

AFP: alpha fetoprotein

AIH: autoimmune hepatitis

ALD: alcoholic liver disease

ALT: alanine aminotransferase

AMA: antimitochondrial antibodies

AST: aspartate aminotransferase

ATD: α_1 antitrypsin deficiency

BMI: body mass index

CT: computed tomography

DILD: drug-induced liver disease

EVL: endoscopic variceal ligation

ES: endoscopic sclerotherapy

GGT: gamma-glutamyltransferase

HBeAg/Ab: hepatitis B 'e' antigen/antibody

HBsAg/Ab: hepatitis B 'surface' antigen/antibody

HBV: hepatitis B virus

HCC: hepatocellular carcinoma

HCV: hepatitis C virus

HELLP: hemolysis, elevated liver enzymes, low platelet count

HFE: High Fe (gene – mutations result in hemochromatosis)

Ig: immunoglobulin

INR: international normalized ratio

LDLT: living donor liver transplant

LVP: large-volume paracentesis

MELD: model for end-stage liver disease

NAFLD: non-alcoholic fatty liver disease

NASH: non-alcoholic steatohepatitis

5NT: 5'nucleotidase

pANCA: perinuclear antineutrophil cytoplasmic antibody

PCR: polymerase chain reaction

PELD: pediatric end-stage liver disease

PiZZ: protease inhibitor, Z variant, homozygous (a mutation of the α_1 antitrypsin gene)

PBC: primary biliary cirrhosis

PSC: primary sclerosing cholangitis

PT: prothrombin time

PTLD: post-transplant lymphoproliferative disease

SAAG: serum–ascites albumin gradient

SBP: spontaneous bacterial peritonitis

TIPS: transjugular intrahepatic portosystemic shunt

TNF: tumor necrosis factor

UDCA: ursodeoxycholic acid

WBC: white blood cell

Introduction

Our aim in this book is to provide a succinct and useful guide to the clinical management of patients with liver disease. Acute presentations of liver disease are common and most resolve spontaneously. However, establishing an accurate diagnosis and understanding the indicators of severe disease are very important in order to avoid delay in identifying the small cohort in need of referral for specialist treatment.

Alcoholic liver disease presents in many forms, and there is an emerging epidemic of similar disease in non-alcohol consumers, particularly related to obesity. Recognition of chronic hepatitis B and C is improving, with more patients receiving antiviral therapy. This is a particularly dynamic area with new therapies emerging quite regularly. The review of these topics is pitched at understanding the most important issues within these chronic liver diseases.

Increasing numbers of patients are undergoing liver function tests and ultrasonic evaluation of the liver, resulting in the identification of abnormalities that need to be put into perspective. We have given this clinical scenario considerable attention, as we believe that in this situation quick access to a common-sense approach to investigation or a simple explanation will be of benefit.

At the other end of the spectrum, many non-specialists and primary care physicians are encountering patients who have been recipients of liver transplants. We deal with some of the commoner associated clinical problems that may need attention in the community.

We hope that you will find this book helpful.

Liver disorders are encountered frequently in general practice. Recent data suggest that 5.5 million Americans have chronic liver disease. At least 1% of asymptomatic patients will have elevated liver test results, although the incidence of abnormal results varies considerably with the population studied. The goals of the physician's investigation are to understand the origin of the liver injury, to correct its cause and to prevent permanent organ dysfunction (i.e. cirrhosis). An organized approach to investigating liver abnormalities allows the physician to reach conclusions promptly, and avoids excessive cost or risk to the patient.

Acute liver injuries

Acute liver injuries are defined by hepatologists as those that resolve within 6 months. Patients with acute liver disease typically have no previous history of liver injury. They may complain of fatigue, anorexia, malaise and discomfort in the right upper quadrant of the abdomen. Jaundice may be seen and tender hepatomegaly elicited. Acute liver injuries (e.g. viral hepatitis, exposure to a toxin or medication) typically resolve once the offending agent is removed or the viral infection resolves, and usually there are no sequelae. Occasionally, however, liver injury is so severe that the patient does not have enough hepatocytes remaining to allow for homeostasis – a condition called fulminant hepatic failure or acute liver failure (see page 20).

Chronic liver injuries

The primary care provider more often encounters chronic, rather than acute, liver disease. Patients typically present with few symptoms, and diagnosis is on the basis of abnormal blood results on routine examination. They may complain of fatigue and malaise. The examiner may find stigmata of chronic liver disease, such as gynecomastia, spider nevi, telangiectasia and palmar erythema. The liver is usually enlarged and may be firm; a tender liver is uncommon. If advanced liver disease has developed (e.g. cirrhosis), signs of portal hypertension, such as caput medusae or ascites, may be present.

History

As with all medical conditions, it is vital to obtain a thorough and accurate history. With respect to liver disease, it is necessary to determine if there is any history of jaundice. Risk factors for viral hepatitis include prior transfusion, multiple sexual partners, tattoo application and needle sharing. Alcohol, of course, is a common hepatic toxin, and physicians must be adept at determining a patient's alcohol consumption. Unfortunately, this is significantly more difficult to accomplish in practice than in theory. Alcoholism is a disease of denial, and many patients will not admit to, or even realize, how much alcohol they consume.

Medications may also cause liver disease, so it is important to determine which medications a patient is taking, and particularly those temporally related to the development of the liver disorder. Some over-the-counter medications and herbal remedies have also been reported to cause liver abnormalities. Although most hepatic toxins are no longer common in the workplace, an occupational history may reveal relevant exposures.

A family history of liver disease is equally important. In our experience the liver disease that most commonly clusters in a family is alcoholic liver disease (ALD), but other diseases such as Wilson's disease and hemochromatosis (see Chapter 6, Metabolic liver diseases) should be considered.

Liver tests

Liver enzymes. The liver typically responds to injury by releasing enzymes from hepatocytes and/or biliary epithelium. Elevated levels of enzymes of hepatocellular origin, such as aspartate aminotransferase (AST) and alanine aminotransferase (ALT), suggest injury to hepatocytes. Elevations in alkaline phosphatase suggest injury to structures of the biliary tree.

AST is a mitochondrial enzyme found in the liver and other tissues, such as skeletal and myocardial muscle. ALT is a cytoplasmic enzyme found primarily in the liver. Both AST and ALT are released from injured hepatocytes, and elevated levels are found in the blood of patients with liver disease of diverse etiologies. In most liver disorders, ALT is higher than AST. When AST is higher than ALT (particularly if the ratio is greater than 2), ALD is strongly suspected.

Elevations of aminotransferases do not necessarily correlate with the severity of liver injury. For example, in severe alcoholic hepatitis, aminotransferases may be no greater than four or five times the upper limit of normal, whereas in asymptomatic acute viral hepatitis, aminotransferase elevations can easily range from 20 to 100 times the upper limit of normal.

Alkaline phosphatase catalyzes phosphatase reactions in alkaline environments in vitro, but its function in vivo is not well defined. However, it has long been established that injury to the bile ducts, whether the extrahepatic bile ducts or the microscopic canaliculi that course through the liver, results in elevated alkaline phosphatase levels in the blood. Alkaline phosphatase is not unique to the liver; it is also found in bone, and to a lesser extent in the placenta and intestine. Identifying which organ is releasing alkaline phosphatase is not particularly difficult, however.

- Patients with elevated alkaline phosphatase of hepatic origin usually have symptoms or signs of liver disease or other hepatic abnormalities on biochemical screening.
- In contrast, patients with elevated alkaline phosphatase of bone origin may complain of bone pain or may be diagnosed with Paget's disease.

On occasion, however, elevated alkaline phosphatase is discovered as an isolated abnormality. In this case, further laboratory tests are required to determine the origin of the alkaline phosphatase. The enzyme 5'nucleotidase (5NT) parallels alkaline phosphatase of hepatic origin. Thus, in liver disease, both the 5NT and the alkaline phosphatase will be elevated, whereas in bone disease 5NT levels will be normal. Likewise, gamma-glutamyltransferase (GGT) parallels alkaline phosphatase of hepatic origin and is normal in bone disease. GGT levels can also be useful in the diagnosis of ALD, as GGT is rapidly inducible by alcohol and often reaches impressive elevations in patients with even mild alcoholic liver injury. As with the aminotransferases, alkaline phosphatase levels do not necessarily correlate with the severity of liver injury or dysfunction. Prothrombin time (PT) and albumin and bilirubin levels are better measures of liver function.

Prothrombin time (PT). All of the clotting factors, with the exception of factor VIII, are produced by the liver. Thus, measurement of PT is a reliable marker of liver function. Because the clotting proteins require vitamin K as a cofactor, vitamin K deficiency must be ruled out as a cause of an increased PT. Parenteral administration of vitamin K to patients with vitamin K deficiency usually corrects the PT within 12–24 hours, whereas vitamin K has a negligible effect in liver failure. Occasionally, vitamin K deficiency and liver disease coincide. With cholestatic liver disorders, such as primary biliary cirrhosis and primary sclerosing cholangitis, the absorption of fat-soluble vitamins such as vitamin K can be impaired. Thus, administering vitamin K to a patient with an elevated PT is reasonable. However, repeated daily injections of vitamin K when there is no apparent improvement in PT are not helpful.

Albumin is a protein synthesized only in the liver. Thus, measurement of the albumin concentration is a reasonable test of the synthetic capacity of the liver. It should be noted, however, that albumin lost through the urine (e.g. nephrotic syndrome) or through the gastrointestinal tract (e.g. inflammatory bowel disease) could mimic hypoalbuminemia of liver origin. Similarly, a patient who is malnourished may not deliver enough substrate to the liver for adequate synthesis of albumin. Malnutrition and liver disease frequently coexist.

Bilirubin. Measurement of the serum bilirubin concentration is perhaps the most important test of liver function. Bilirubin is a product of the turnover of red blood cells, with a relatively constant value in the serum. Hyperbilirubinemia signifies one of several scenarios.

- An increased load of bilirubin may be delivered to the liver from the periphery, as occurs in hemolysis. Review of the peripheral smear or measurement of lactate dehydrogenase or haptoglobin helps to eliminate hemolysis as a cause of increased bilirubin levels.
- Injury of liver cells (e.g. in hepatitis or cirrhosis) is another possible cause of elevated bilirubin levels. Substantial hepatocellular injury prevents water-insoluble unconjugated (indirect) bilirubin from being conjugated with glucuronic acid to form its water-soluble conjugated (direct) form. Thus, both acute and chronic liver disease may result in elevation of the serum bilirubin level because of injury to or loss of hepatocytes.
- Obstruction to bile flow, which can occur anywhere along the biliary tree from the microscopic canaliculi to the large extrahepatic bile ducts, can also lead to elevated serum bilirubin. Obstruction may result from physical abnormalities, such as a stone resting in the common bile duct or a tumor in the pancreas, that physically prevent bilirubin from exiting the liver. More subtle insults can also occur, such as injuries to the microscopic biliary canaliculi by medications such as estrogen and chlorpromazine.
- Sepsis may cause dysfunction of the mechanism of bilirubin transport across the canalicular membrane, leading to hyperbilirubinemia.
- Inherited disorders of bilirubin metabolism may result in increased serum bilirubin levels. Gilbert's syndrome is the most common of these, affecting approximately 4% of the population. Gilbert's syndrome results from a mutation in the gene that controls the production of uridine diphosphate glucuronosyltransferase, the enzyme that conjugates bilirubin from its water-insoluble to its water-soluble form. Thus, these patients have elevations of unconjugated (indirect) bilirubin levels. An important clue to the diagnosis of Gilbert's syndrome is otherwise normal liver function; albumin concentration, PT, aminotransferases and alkaline phosphatase are all normal. These patients require only reassurance.

Imaging and biopsy
Radiology plays an important role in the evaluation of patients with some forms of liver disease. Ultrasonography is particularly useful for

examining the hepatic parenchyma for abnormalities (e.g. tumors or other space-occupying lesions) and the biliary tree for dilation induced by distal obstruction. Increased echo texture is usually interpreted as a sign of fatty infiltration of the liver or hepatocellular unrest, such as that which accompanies viral hepatitis. It is our opinion, however, that this is neither sensitive nor specific, and findings must be interpreted in the overall clinical context.

Computed tomography (CT) can identify space-occupying lesions measuring more than 1 cm. In addition, fatty infiltration of the liver can be diagnosed with reasonable sensitivity and specificity. CT also provides good views of the biliary tree, pancreas and other intra-abdominal organs.

A liver biopsy is the gold standard for evaluation of liver disease. Although patients approach biopsy with trepidation, it is safe and quite simple to perform. Most liver biopsies are now performed under ultrasound guidance on an outpatient basis. Generally, a biopsy is safe provided that the PT is prolonged by no more than a few seconds and the platelet count is greater than $70\ 000 \times 10^{-6}$/L. A liver biopsy usually allows a definitive diagnosis of the underlying liver disorder and staging of the disease (severity of permanent liver injury; fibrosis; cirrhosis).

Investigational pathways for mildly abnormal liver function tests

Mild elevations in AST, ALT and GGT are commonly detected on programmed health evaluations or during the investigation of unrelated symptoms. An elevated GGT level is particularly common, with levels up to five times the upper limit of normal, usually with a lesser degree of abnormality in alkaline phosphatase. The serum aminotransferases (transaminase) may be normal or increased to 4–5 times the upper limit of normal. The serum bilirubin and albumin and PT are normal.

The initial evaluation is:
- take a history of alcohol usage
- elicit drug exposure during the previous 6 months
- screen for diabetes or family history of diabetes
- weigh, and calculate the body mass index (BMI).

Regular alcohol use can account for this pattern of abnormal liver function tests, even if the intake is not considered excessive. This particularly applies to women. Elevated mean corpuscular volume provides strong supporting evidence that alcohol is the underlying cause. A trial of abstinence from alcohol for 3 months will determine the contribution of alcohol to the abnormality (an algorithm for investigations is shown in Figure 1.1).

Non-alcoholic fatty liver disease and non-alcoholic steatohepatitis are equally common explanations for this pattern of abnormal liver function tests. The diagnosis is more likely against the background of:

- credible history of minimal or no alcohol consumption
- increased BMI or obesity
- non-insulin-dependent diabetes mellitus or family history of diabetes
- hyperlipidemia, particularly hypertriglyceridemia.

An ultrasound examination will detect fatty infiltration in many cases, but its absence does not exclude the possible diagnosis of fatty liver and it will not differentiate between non-alcoholic fatty liver disease and alcohol-related fatty liver.

The liver function profile may underestimate the severity of the liver disease in a minority of patients. A liver biopsy should be performed if

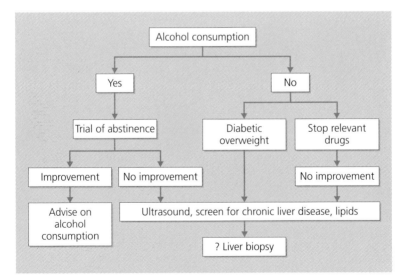

Figure 1.1 Investigational pathway for mild elevations in aspartate aminotransferase, alanine aminotransferase and gamma-glutamyltransferase.

there are any indicators of portal hypertension (e.g. platelet count below normal or an enlarged spleen on ultrasonography).

Isolated increase in aminotransferases. Serum aminotransferases may be mildly increased in association with a range of innocuous intercurrent infections. A solitary finding does not warrant immediate extensive investigation (Figure 1.2) unless a risk factor for chronic viral hepatitis is identified, such as:
• ethnic background associated with high risk
• intravenous drug use at any period of life
• receipt of blood products before 1990
• tattoos
• homosexual activity or known sexual exposure.
In other instances, liver function tests should be repeated after about 3 months and investigations performed if the abnormality persists. Screening for chronic viral hepatitis B and C is the most critical part of the evaluation. When the viral screen is negative, investigations

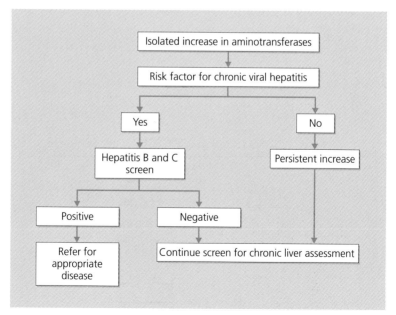

Figure 1.2 Investigational pathway for isolated increases in liver aminotransferases.

should be extended to cover other causes of chronic liver disease and include:

- autoantibody screen
- immunoglobulin measurements
- ceruloplasmin measurement
- ferritin measurement
- determination of α_1 antitrypsin phenotype.

An ultrasound scan of the liver and possibly a liver biopsy complete the investigation in most instances.

Isolated increased serum bilirubin as the only abnormality in the liver function profile is usually due to Gilbert's syndrome, a congenital abnormality that occurs in 4% of the population. The bilirubin is predominantly unconjugated. The main differential diagnosis is chronic hemolytic anemia (e.g. due to spherocytosis). The bilirubin increases during intercurrent illnesses and, as a result, the patient may inappropriately attribute the associated symptoms to being jaundiced. Gilbert's syndrome is entirely innocuous.

Key points – investigating liver disease

- Elevated levels of aspartate aminotransferase and alanine aminotransferase suggest injury to hepatocytes.
- An elevated level of alkaline phosphatase suggests injury to structures of the biliary tree.
- Prothrombin time (after vitamin K) and serum albumin are used to assess the liver's ability to synthesize proteins.
- Increases in serum bilirubin occur for many reasons, but generally indicate severe disease.
- At least 1% of asymptomatic individuals have abnormal liver function test results.

Key references

American Gastroenterological Association. Medical position statement: evaluation of liver chemistry tests. *Gastroenterology* 2002;123:1364–6.

American Gastroenterological Association. Technical review on the evaluation of liver chemistry tests. *Gastroenterology* 2002;123: 1367–84.

Ben-Menachem DS, Vasudevan G, Ma CK, Blumenkehl M. Prospective evaluation on unexplained chronic liver transaminase abnormalities in asymptomatic and symptomatic patients. *Am J Gastroenterol* 1999; 94:3010–14.

Gopal DV, Rosen HR. Abnormal findings on liver function tests. Interpreting results to narrow the diagnosis and establish a prognosis. *Postgrad Med* 2002;107:100–14.

Johnston DE. Special considerations in interpreting liver function tests. *Am Fam Physician* 199;59:2223–30.

Pratt DS, Kaplan MM. Evaluation of abnormal liver-enzyme results in asymptomatic patients. *N Engl J Med* 2000;342:1266–71.

Sorbi D, McGill DB, Thistle JL et al. An assessment of the role of liver biopsies in asymptomatic patients with chronic liver test abnormalities. *Am J Gastroenterol* 2000;95: 3206–10.

Acute liver disease refers to diseases of less than 6 months' duration at the time of presentation. This category of disease excludes first presentations of cirrhosis, with a few exceptions, such as when hepatitis B or Wilson's disease present with the syndrome of acute liver failure. There are three major categories of acute liver disease:

- hepatitis
- cholestasis
- vascular disease.

The associated symptoms and biochemical profiles differentiate between these patterns of disease (Table 2.1). Jaundice is the typical presentation

TABLE 2.1

Characteristics of the main presentations of acute liver disease

	Hepatitis	Cholestasis	Vascular
Jaundice	Common	Common	Mild
Dark urine	Yes	Yes	No
Pale feces	Unusual	Yes	No
Itch	Unusual	Yes	No
Ascites	Unusual	No	Yes
Serum bilirubin	Variable but may be high	Variable but may be high	< 100 μmol/L (< 6 mg/dL)
Aminotransferases	> 500 IU/L but often much higher	< 300 IU/L	Usually < 300 IU/L
Cholestatic enzymes	Usually < 3 × normal	High	Usually < 2 × normal
Albumin	Normal	Normal	Normal or low
Significance of coagulopathy	Risk of acute liver failure	Vitamin K deficiency	Risk of acute liver failure

of both hepatitis and cholestasis; the sudden onset of ascites is the most common presentation of vascular disease.

Hepatitis

Viral infections and drug reactions account for most cases of acute hepatitis with an identifiable cause (Table 2.2). The liver function profile reveals a predominant increase in the serum aminotransferases (transaminases), with figures in excess of 1000 IU/L in the early phase. The serum bilirubin level increases as the aminotransferase levels fall. The severity of the acute hepatitis is reflected in three clinical categories:

- uncomplicated hepatitis
- severe hepatitis
- acute liver failure.

The development of a coagulopathy (prolonged prothrombin time [PT] or international normalized ratio [INR], reduced factor V levels)

TABLE 2.2

Causes of acute hepatitis

Viral	Drugs
• Hepatitis A	• Dose-dependent: acetaminophen (paracetamol)
• Hepatitis B (occasionally with hepatitis D)	
• Hepatitis E	• Idiosyncratic (e.g. isoniazid, amiodarone, phenytoin, non-steroidal anti-inflammatory drugs, Ecstacy)
• Seronegative or indeterminate hepatitis	
• Leptospirosis (Weil's disease)	
• Rare	**Other causes**
– hepatitis C	• Autoimmune hepatitis
– herpes simplex	• Ischemia
– cytomegalovirus	
– Epstein–Barr virus	
– adenovirus	

determines the transition to severe hepatitis. The onset of acute liver failure is signaled by the onset of encephalopathy (a neurological syndrome ranging in severity from drowsiness and poor concentration to coma).

Acute hepatitis has a prodromal phase, during which anorexia, nausea, vomiting and loss of appetite for food and cigarettes are typical features. The prodromal phase is as short as 1 week for hepatitis A but may be as long as 3 months for hepatitis B. This is usually followed by the onset of jaundice, although this is not always the case in young children. The prodromal symptoms characteristically improve once jaundice develops. The jaundice resolves over variable periods but usually within 6 weeks of onset. Lethargy may be profound and persist for months after the jaundice has cleared.

Hepatitis A is contracted by the orofecal route. Childhood exposure is now the norm only in developing countries; accordingly, in the Western world, immunity levels in teenagers have fallen to below 5%. Childhood infection usually causes a non-specific illness; the likelihood of developing jaundice increases with age at acquisition. Adults may acquire hepatitis from infected water or shellfish, travel to endemic areas or occupational or sexual exposure.

Hepatitis A is one of the few causes of acute hepatitis that results in fever. The risk of developing acute liver failure is only 0.1% overall, increasing exponentially with age. Hepatitis is a biphasic illness in 6–10% of cases and is followed by a cholestatic phase in about 5%. There is no specific treatment for hepatitis A, and it does not have a chronic carrier state in humans. Vaccination against hepatitis A is effective and is advised for travelers to endemic areas, individuals at occupational risk, patients with chronic liver disease and homosexual men.

Hepatitis B is contracted by vertical transmission, sexual exposure and contact with infected blood. Vertical transmission occurs at birth and is the main route of infection in highly endemic areas. Chronic carriage follows neonatal exposure in 95% of cases, whereas only 5% of adults who contract hepatitis B become chronic carriers. Patients with acute hepatitis B are increasingly being treated with antiviral agents such as lamivudine and adefovir. Vaccination is effective in preventing infection in over 95% of individuals. Target populations for vaccination include healthcare workers and homosexual men.

Seronegative or indeterminate hepatitis are two of the terms used to describe a presumed viral hepatitis for which no cause can be identified. This entity occurs particularly in patients developing acute liver failure. Although assumed to be viral, this condition has a propensity for middle-aged women and does not occur in clusters. Unrecognized toxins or autoimmune processes are alternative explanations. A suppressed history of recreational Ecstacy use is worth considering in young patients with this clinical picture.

Hepatitis C and E. Hepatitis C is rarely identified as a cause of acute hepatitis. Hepatitis E is common in the Indian subcontinent, and sporadic cases are being identified increasingly in the West. The natural history is similar to that of hepatitis A. However, hepatitis E is associated with a peculiarly high mortality in pregnant women. There is no effective vaccine for hepatitis C or hepatitis E.

Leptospirosis or Weil's disease is an unusual cause of acute hepatitis, typically acquired by contact with rat's urine. Rapid diagnosis is important because of the potential for effective treatment with penicillin in the early phase. Characteristic features include fever, hemorrhagic skin rash and renal dysfunction.

Other causes. Idiosyncratic reactions leading to hepatitis may follow exposure to a wide range of drugs; some of the more common causes are listed in Table 2.2.

Autoimmune hepatitis may present for the first time with an episode of florid hepatitis.

Acute liver failure

Acute liver failure is a life-threatening complication of acute hepatitis and a number of other liver diseases (Wilson's disease, acute fatty liver of pregnancy, Budd–Chiari syndrome and *Amanita phalloides* mushroom poisoning). The definition of acute liver failure is based on the development of encephalopathy within 12 weeks of the onset of jaundice. Hypoglycemia may mimic encephalopathy, but its occurrence is an independent indicator of severe liver injury and risk of later progression to encephalopathy. A coagulopathy is invariably present. PT rises and the bilirubin rockets upwards. Many of these patients will die unless they receive a liver transplant.

Acute liver failure causes multi-system failure (Figure 2.1).

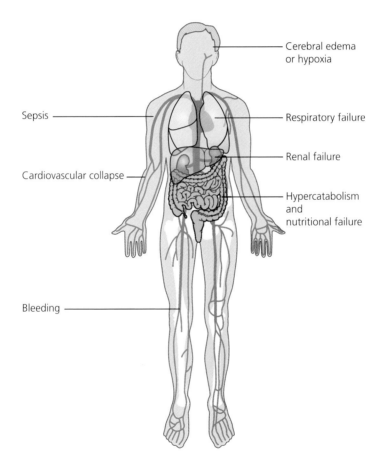

Figure 2.1 Complications of acute liver failure, leading to multi-system failure.

Neurological complications are a major cause of death, as a result of either severe cerebral hypoxia or brainstem herniation complicating cerebral edema. Sepsis and circulatory failure account for most other deaths. The development of renal failure also indicates a poorer prognosis. Overall, about 30% of patients survive without surgery, 40% undergo emergency liver transplantation, with survival rates of 70–80%, and the remaining 30% die. Specific prognostic models are used in specialist centers to determine prognosis and the need for liver transplantation. Outcome is heavily influenced by the underlying etiology, the age of the patient and the rate of progression of the disease. A number of easily recognizable scenarios that are associated with either a favorable or unfavorable outcome are given in Table 2.3.

TABLE 2.3

Features suggestive of a favorable or unfavorable outcome in acute liver failure

Favorable

- Acetaminophen (paracetamol) overdose with no evidence of metabolic acidosis or renal failure, despite the presence of a severe coagulopathy
- Pregnancy-related syndromes
- Viral hepatitis A or B, encephalopathy developing within 7 days of onset of jaundice

Unfavorable

- Seronegative hepatitis or idiosyncratic drug reactions
- Wilson's disease
- Encephalopathy developing more than 7 days after onset of jaundice
- Jaundice for more than 4 weeks despite coagulopathy and encephalopathy being mild
- Young children
- Adults over 40 years of age
- Acetaminophen overdose with severe metabolic acidosis or combination of severe encephalopathy, renal failure and severe coagulopathy

Acetaminophen (paracetamol) overdose induces a distinct pattern of acute liver failure. Acidosis may be an early feature, and failure to reverse the acidosis within 24 hours of drug ingestion is associated with a very high mortality. Patients at risk of acute liver failure are identified by the development of a coagulopathy, and encephalopathy typically develops on the third or fourth day after the overdose. Renal failure is more common, and occurs earlier than with other causes of acute liver failure. Progression to acute liver failure is usually prevented by the administration of N-acetylcysteine within 16–24 hours of the overdose. Later administration of N-acetylcysteine may also modify the severity of the disease.

Wilson's disease, an inherited disorder of copper metabolism, may present with many of the clinical features of acute liver failure. It is therefore classified as acute, even though the majority of patients have cirrhosis at the time of presentation. Hemolytic anemia and ascites early in the course of the disease are characteristics of Wilson's disease.

Cholestasis

Cholestatic jaundice is characterized predominantly by elevations in alkaline phosphatase and gamma-glutamyltransferase (GGT). Most cases are caused by extrahepatic biliary obstruction (Table 2.4). The presence of pain points to gallstone disease; conversely, the absence of pain suggests malignant disease, especially in older patients. Biliary obstruction causes dilation of the bile ducts and is easily detected on ultrasound examination, which is the initial screening procedure. More precise definition of the site of the obstruction is then obtained by endoscopic or magnetic resonance cholangiography.

Intrahepatic causes of cholestasis are considered when there is no evidence of duct dilation on ultrasound examination. Jaundice and pruritus are the dominant clinical features. The urine is dark in color, the stools are pale and weight loss may be considerable. The liver function profile confirms elevated serum bilirubin, serum alkaline phosphatase and GGT, but there are no features distinguishing intrahepatic from extrahepatic biliary obstruction. There may be an abnormality in coagulation tests in protracted cases, but this is corrected

TABLE 2.4

Causes of extrahepatic biliary obstruction

- Gallstones
- Cholangiocarcinoma
  - hilar
  - mid or lower bile duct
- Ampullary adenocarcinoma
- Adenocarcinoma of the head of the pancreas
- Benign inflammatory stricture
- Postsurgical stricture (particularly after laparoscopic cholecystectomy)
- Primary sclerosing cholangitis, with or without complicating cholangiocarcinoma

rapidly by parenteral administration of vitamin K. There is no specific therapy other than symptomatic relief, particularly of the pruritus – colestyramine (cholestyramine), ursodeoxycholic acid, rifampin (rifampicin). The duration of the cholestatic episode is variable but it can last for many months.

Cholestasis may be caused by an idiosyncratic drug reaction (Table 2.5). Drug-induced cholestasis is likely to recur with repeated exposure to the offending agent. Cholestasis induced by estrogen in contraceptive pills indicates a high risk of developing cholestasis during subsequent pregnancies.

Benign recurrent cholestasis is a poorly understood entity of recurring episodes of cholestasis without an obvious precipitating cause.

Cholestasis may also be caused by injury to small bile ducts (e.g. as a manifestation of flucloxacillin hepatotoxicity).

Cholestasis may herald Hodgkin's lymphoma as a paraneoplastic syndrome.

Vascular disease

Hepatic vein thrombosis, or Budd–Chiari syndrome, may have an acute presentation with abdominal pain and massive ascites. The liver

TABLE 2.5

Drugs associated with cholestatic reactions

- Estrogens and androgens
- Chlorpromazine
- Tricyclic antidepressants
- Barbiturates
- Phenytoin
- Amitriptyline
- Carbamazepine
- Erythromycin
- Flucloxacillin

function profile shows modest elevation in the serum bilirubin and aminotransferases. A coagulopathy indicates that the liver insult is severe and the patient is at risk of acute liver failure. Most cases have an underlying procoagulant state that may be occult. The most frequent associations are:

- factor V Leiden
- antiphospholipid antibody syndrome
- essential thrombocythemia
- polycythemia rubra vera
- antithrombin III deficiency
- protein C or S deficiency
- paroxysmal nocturnal hemoglobinuria.

Mechanical obstruction with cysts or tumors may precipitate the thrombosis; in Asians from the Far East, webs in the vena cava are a notable cause of Budd–Chiari syndrome.

The diagnosis is suggested by failure to demonstrate patent hepatic veins on ultrasonography or computed tomography scanning and is confirmed by direct venography. A liver biopsy may be useful in identifying long-standing cases, and may reveal significant fibrosis or cirrhosis. The usual treatment of acute Budd–Chiari syndrome is a decompressive shunt, fashioned either surgically or by construction of a

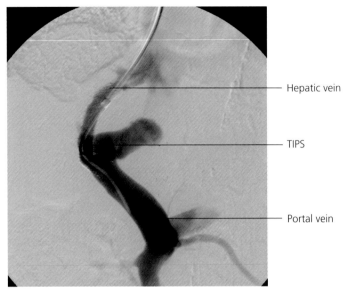

Hepatic vein

TIPS

Portal vein

Figure 2.2 Transjugular intrahepatic portosystemic shunt (TIPS) immediately after insertion, with catheter still in situ.

transjugular intrahepatic portosystemic shunt (TIPS) (Figure 2.2). Liver transplantation is indicated in patients with established cirrhosis, those showing manifestations of acute liver failure and those whose condition deteriorates after shunting.

Veno-occlusive disease is clinically similar to the Budd–Chiari syndrome, but the main hepatic veins are patent and the obstruction occurs in the small hepatic venules. The disease may be caused by alkaloids (e.g. those present in bush tea and some chemotherapeutic agents); it also occurs after bone marrow transplantation. Management is similar to that of Budd–Chiari syndrome.

Key points – acute liver disease

- Attempt to classify acute liver disease as hepatitis (most common), cholestatic (intermediate) or vascular (unusual).
- Simple blood tests and an ultrasound examination provide most of the information required.
- Hypoglycemia, coagulopathy and any evidence of confusion indicate a high risk of acute liver failure and the need for specialist care.
- Coagulopathy in cholestatic disorders responds to parenteral vitamin K.

Key references

Lake JR, Sussman NL. Determining prognosis in patients with fulminant hepatic failure: when you absolutely, positively have to know the answer. *Hepatology* 1995;21:879–82.

Norris S. Drug- and toxin-induced liver damage. In: O'Grady JG, Lake JR, Howdle PD, eds. *Comprehensive Clinical Hepatology*. London: Mosby, 2000:ch 29.1, pp 1–20.

Valla D-C. The diagnosis and management of the Budd–Chiari syndrome: consensus and controversies. *Hepatology* 2003;38:793–803.

Alcoholic liver disease (ALD) is a common cause of end-stage liver disease, resulting in substantial morbidity and mortality throughout the world. In the USA, approximately 2 million people suffer from an alcohol-induced liver disorder. Medical costs associated with caring for these patients are enormous. Alcohol-related liver injury presents a spectrum of disease, including asymptomatic hepatic steatosis (fatty liver), steatosis accompanied by inflammation (steatohepatitis or alcoholic hepatitis), cirrhosis with liver failure, variceal bleeding, ascites and even the development of hepatocellular carcinoma. Early intervention for patients presenting with the early stages of liver injury helps to prevent further, permanent liver injury. Interrupting alcoholism is the key, but this is not an easy task and frustrates many primary care providers, families and patients.

Presentation

Patients may present anywhere along the spectrum of ALD. Those with steatosis only usually have few symptoms or signs of liver disease and are typically identified only by abnormal liver tests. Patients with alcoholic hepatitis are usually jaundiced and report fatigue, malaise and anorexia. The liver is enlarged and tender, and ascites and edema are often present. Patients with established cirrhosis usually display signs of portal hypertension, such as splenomegaly, caput medusae and ascites. In late-stage disease, the liver may be small and hard and there may be cutaneous stigmata of chronic liver disease, such as palmar erythema, spider nevi or telangiectasia. Gynecomastia and small shrunken testicles may be present in men. Diagnosis and treatment are summarized in Table 3.1.

Liver function tests. Examination of laboratory results is helpful in diagnosing ALD. The aminotransferases are elevated and have a characteristic pattern in patients with ALD: the aspartate aminotransferase (AST) is almost always higher than the alanine

TABLE 3.1

Diagnosis and treatment of alcoholic liver disease

Alcoholic steatosis	Alcoholic hepatitis	Alcoholic cirrhosis
Symptoms		
Few, non-specific	Malaise, nausea, fatigue	Variable
Examination		
Hepatomegaly	Hepatomegaly, jaundice, ascites	Cutaneous stigmata of liver disease, portal hypertension
Laboratory tests		
AST > ALT, normal bilirubin, albumin and PT, GGT elevated	AST > ALT, WBCs elevated, bilirubin elevated, albumin depressed	PT elevated, bilirubin elevated, albumin depressed, platelet count low
Histology		
Steatosis	Steatosis with active inflammation	Fibrosis
Treatment		
Abstinence	Abstinence; aggressive nutrition, consider glucocorticoids	Abstinence; treat complications

ALT, alanine aminotransferase; AST, aspartate aminotransferase; GGT, gamma-glutamyltransferase; PT, prothrombin time; WBC, white blood cell.

aminotransferase (ALT) level, and the greater the ratio, the more likely that the liver disease is due to alcohol. In liver disease of non-alcoholic etiology, the ALT is typically higher than the AST. Alkaline phosphatase and serum bilirubin levels may be increased, the prothrombin time prolonged, and the albumin level depressed. The latter are good markers of the severity of ALD. However, it should also be noted that liver function tests may be entirely normal in the presence of cirrhosis.

Further investigations. Ultrasound or computed tomography images of the abdomen typically show parenchymal abnormalities suggestive of fatty changes in the liver, and may show a nodular outline typical of cirrhosis. Changes of portal hypertension, such as portosystemic collaterals and ascites, can also be seen on imaging studies. A liver biopsy is the gold standard for diagnosing ALD and in documenting the severity of liver injury, but may not be required in all cases. This is particularly true when the patient's history is suggestive of ALD, there is no evidence of viral hepatitis and biopsy could be difficult (i.e. patients with coagulopathy or severe ascites).

Concomitant disease. It is important to rule out other forms of liver disease and to document any concomitant injurious agents. Chronic hepatitis C and, to a lesser extent, hepatitis B are common in patients with alcoholism. Although most patients who drink alcohol never develop significant liver disease, and many patients with viral hepatitis do well over long periods of time, the combination of viral hepatitis and alcoholism often accelerates the development of advanced liver injury. Thus, identification of a patient with both diseases is important.

There is an interesting parallel between ALD and the more recently recognized non-alcoholic fatty liver disease (NAFLD; see Chapter 6, Metabolic liver diseases), which is usually seen in patients with insulin resistance, obesity or diabetes. Both disorders are characterized by the deposition of fat (triglyceride) in the liver and progression through stages of inflammation to collagen deposition and fibrosis. Histologically, ALD and NAFLD appear identical, and some investigators feel that they differ only in the mechanism by which fat is originally deposited. Once fat appears in the liver, a similar progression of events occurs, resulting in irreversible scarring in the liver.

Determination of alcohol consumption. Although it seems self-evident, the diagnosis of ALD is made easier if it can be documented that the patient is drinking injurious amounts of alcohol (i.e. 80 g – about six drinks – per day for men and as little as 20 g per day for women). Accurate determination of alcohol consumption can be difficult, however, as patients often under-report how much alcohol they consume, and denial is common. The CAGE questionnaire, the Alcohol Use Disorders Identification Test and reports from families may be helpful in identifying patients whose alcohol consumption is excessive. It should be remembered, however, that small amounts of alcohol (1–2 drinks per day) are probably beneficial, as has been reported extensively in the medical literature and popularized by the lay press. Small amounts of alcohol would not be expected to cause ALD in men and, if it can be confirmed that a patient consumes only a small amount of alcohol, other causes of liver disease must be considered.

Treatment

The treatment of ALD essentially entails abstinence from alcohol, which is clearly the most important factor in promoting both short- and long-term survival. Achieving abstinence typically requires a multidisciplinary approach, involving organizations such as Alcoholics Anonymous, professional alcoholism counselors and, often, mental health professionals. This requires a substantial commitment on the part of the patient and the patient's family. Ideally, the patient will be encouraged by the knowledge that, with cessation of alcohol intake, their liver function is likely to improve substantially.

Nutrition. Alcoholics are usually malnourished, and improving nutrition is associated with improved outcomes. This is particularly important for patients with alcoholic hepatitis. Anorexia may prevent adequate nutrition and feeding via an enteral tube is often required. Most alcoholics need protein. Unfortunately, however, a few patients with advanced liver disease develop hepatic encephalopathy when given large amounts of protein. Consultation with dietitians may be beneficial, and dietary supplements including protein formulas that are less likely to produce hepatic encephalopathy (branched-chain amino acids) may be helpful.

Corticosteroids. Alcoholic hepatitis is an inflammatory condition. Thus, corticosteroids are a logical treatment for ALD. However, despite many studies that have investigated the role of corticosteroids

---

Key points – alcoholic liver disease

- Alcoholic liver disease (ALD) is a common cause of end-stage liver disease.
- Early intervention prevents permanent injury, but interrupting alcoholism can be difficult.
- Patients with ALD typically have mild to moderate elevations in aminotransferases, with AST > ALT.
- Patients with ALD are often malnourished; improving nutrition is an important treatment goal.
- Patients with severe alcoholic hepatitis may benefit from glucocorticoids or pentoxifylline.

---

in the treatment of alcoholic hepatitis, there is no clear consensus on their efficacy. Most hepatologists believe that the most severe forms of alcoholic hepatitis, and particularly patients with hepatic encephalopathy, benefit from a course of glucocorticoids.

Tumor necrosis factor. Elevated levels of tumor necrosis factor (TNF) have been recorded in patients with alcoholic hepatitis, and clinical outcome appears to correlate with TNF levels. Efforts to decrease TNF levels have shown some promise in the treatment of patients with alcoholic hepatitis. Recent studies have documented that pentoxifylline improved survival in patients with alcoholic hepatitis, presumably by interfering with TNF.

Liver transplantation for patients with ALD remains a controversial topic. Most transplant centers will consider patients with ALD as candidates for transplantation provided they have a documented period of abstinence of at least 6 months before transplantation is considered. Unfortunately, some patients do return to drinking following transplant, although long-term success is common.

Key references

Babor TF, Biddle-Higgins JC, Saunders JB, Monteiro MG. AUDIT: *The Alcohol Use Disorders Identification Test: Guidelines for Use in Primary Health Care*. Geneva: World Health Organization, 2001. http://whqlibdoc.who.int/hq/2001/W HO_MSD_MSB_01.6a.pdf

Ewing JA. Detecting alcoholism: the CAGE questionaire. *JAMA* 1984;252:1905–7.

Fiellin DA, Reid MC, O'Connor PG. Screening for alcohol problems in primary care: a systematic review. *Arch Intern Med* 2000;160:1977–89.

Gordon H. Detection of alcoholic liver disease. *World J Gastroenterol* 2001;7:297–302.

Hoofnagle JH, Kresina T, Fuller RK et al. Liver transplantation for alcoholic liver disease: executive statement and recommendations. Summary of a National Institutes of Health workshop held December 6–7, 1996, Bethesda, Maryland. *Liver Transpl Surg* 1997;3:347–50.

Maher JJ. Treatment of alcoholic hepatitis. *J Gastroenterol Hepatol* 2002;17:448–55.

McCullough AJ, O'Connor JF. Alcoholic liver disease: proposed recommendations for the American College of Gastroenterology. *Am J Gastroenterol* 1998;93:2022–36.

Menon KVN, Gores GJ, Shah VH. Pathogenesis, diagnosis and treatment of alcoholic liver disease. *Mayo Clin Proc* 2001;76Z:1021–9.

The liver is uniquely positioned, both anatomically and metabolically, to receive the brunt of potential insults; thus, medications have the potential to induce liver disease, and at least 1000 drugs have been implicated. Medications appear to be the cause of 50% of cases of acute liver failure in the USA, and as pharmacotherapy advances the treatment of many disorders, drug-induced liver disease (DILD) may also rise. The growing use of herbal preparations is also of great concern. Whereas all approved medications have been evaluated at least superficially for hepatotoxicity, the majority of 'natural' remedies have not.

Prompt recognition of DILD is important because continued use of the drug often results in poor outcome. Unfortunately, other than the use of N-acetylcysteine for acetaminophen (paracetamol)-induced hepatotoxicity, there are no specific 'antidotes' for DILD. Stopping the offending medication, supportive care and, in some circumstances, liver transplantation are the only treatments.

DILD typically presents in one of three clinical patterns (Table 4.1). These presentations are similar or even identical to liver injuries from other causes. Thus, identification of DILD relies more on the history of exposure than on any particular finding on examination or from laboratory investigations. Specific medications typically produce a specific and reproducible pattern of liver injury, referred to as the hepatotoxicity signature of the drug.

Two general pathogenetic mechanisms are recognized.

- Predictable or direct DILD usually promptly follows an exposure to a new medication and appears to be due to direct toxicity or a toxic metabolite. Acetaminophen is an example.
- Unpredictable or idiosyncratic DILD may be related to immune hypersensitivity: rash, fever and eosinophilia are typically present. These reactions follow a few weeks after exposure. Hepatotoxicity due to amoxicillin–clavulonic acid is an example. Late-onset idiosyncratic reactions are difficult to recognize. They follow

TABLE 4.1

Clinical patterns of drug-induced liver disease

Cells injured	Presentation	Examples of causative drugs
Hepatitis-like		
Hepatocytes	Elevated aminotransferases	Acetaminophen, thiazolidinediones (e.g. pioglitazone, isoniazid), statins
Cholestasis		
Biliary canaliculi	Elevated alkaline phosphatase, pruritus	Chlorpromazine, erythromycin, estrogens
Mixed		
Biliary canaliculi and hepatocytes	Variable elevations in aminotransferases and alkaline phosphatase	Amoxicillin– clavulanic acid

exposure by many months and usually do not display features of hypersensitivity. Isoniazid is an example.

Drugs commonly associated with hepatotoxicity

Statins (3-hydroxy-3-methylglutaryl coenzyme A (HMG-CoA) reductase inhibitors) reduce cardiovascular morbidity and mortality in patients with and without cardiovascular disease. These drugs are so effective that their use will expand dramatically over the next several years. As a group the statins are very safe, with fewer than 2% of patients enrolled in clinical trials discontinuing the medications for any reason. Nevertheless, elevation of the aminotransferases (greater than 3 times normal) occurs in approximately 1% of exposed patients. Lesser elevations in the aminotransferases are more common (i.e. about 3%). The effect appears to be dose-related and usually occurs in the first few months of therapy. Most patients are asymptomatic and have no signs suggestive of liver dysfunction on physical examination. Severe liver injury has been reported but is rare. Periodic monitoring of liver tests is recommended – but evidence that monitoring prevents serious liver disease is lacking. The abnormalities are generally not progressive and may resolve despite continued use of the drug. Nevertheless, if significant, persistent elevations in liver tests occur, the statin should be discontinued. Starting a different statin once the liver abnormalities have resolved is appropriate.

A common clinical question is whether to use a statin in a patient with pre-existing liver disease. Unfortunately, there is little evidence on which to make an informed decision. A recent retrospective study found that patients with baseline elevated aminotransferases were no more likely to develop further elevation in liver tests when taking a statin than were patients with abnormal aminotransferases who were not taking statins. Thus, it is probably acceptable to use the statins in patients with chronic stable liver disease, provided symptoms and liver tests are monitored. Statins are contraindicated in patients with acute liver disease and those with advanced chronic liver disease (elevated bilirubin, depressed albumin, clinically apparent cirrhosis, etc.).

Acetaminophen (paracetamol) is a remarkably safe drug, but in certain circumstances it has significant hepatotoxicity.
- Doses greater than approximately 10 g, usually taken as a suicide attempt, are a well-known cause of liver failure.
- Recently it has been recognized that lower doses, typically used without suicidal intent, can induce severe liver injury in patients who chronically use alcohol or who are malnourished. In these patients, doses within the therapeutic range (i.e. about 4 g) may be hepatotoxic.

Although non-specific symptoms such as nausea, vomiting and malaise are common within a few hours, patients typically have little evidence of liver injury until 24–48 hours after ingesting injurious amounts of acetaminophen. The aminotransferases rise, occasionally peaking above 10 000 IU/L, and bilirubin is usually modestly elevated. Prothrombin time (PT), however, is often markedly prolonged. Right upper quadrant abdominal pain and signs of hepatic encephalopathy may develop. Renal failure is often seen. The clinical and laboratory abnormalities usually reach their peak by 3–4 days. For those who survive, recovery is usually prompt and complete and there do not appear to be any long-term sequelae to acute acetaminophen liver injury.

The potential for hepatotoxicity following ingestion can be calculated using the Rumack–Matthew acetaminophen nomogram (Figure 4.1). Serum acetaminophen levels (drawn at least 4 hours after ingestion) are plotted against the time since ingestion. Patients with intersects below the line in the nomogram are at little risk for hepatotoxicity. It should be noted that the Rumack–Matthew nomogram may be inaccurate if overdose is with one of the many extended-release acetaminophen preparations now available.

Treatment. Activated charcoal should be given when the patient presents within 8 hours of ingestion. N-acetylcysteine is the definitive treatment for acetaminophen overdose. It serves as a glutathione precursor, promoting the elimination of N-acetylbenzoquinoneimine, a hepatotoxic metabolite of acetaminophen. Significant hepatotoxicity is uncommon when N-acetylcysteine is given within 8 hours of overdose. It is therefore imperative that N-acetylcysteine is given early (typically

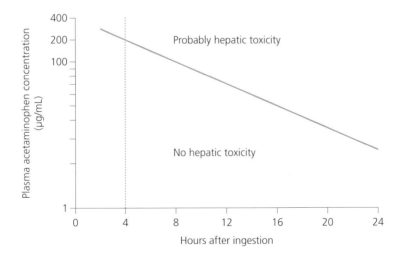

Figure 4.1 The Rumack–Matthew nomogram is used to calculate the potential for hepatotoxicity following ingestion of standard acetaminophen tablets. Reproduced from Rumack and Matthew, 1975.

while awaiting acetaminophen serum levels) and is continued even if significant hepatotoxicity has developed. If the nomogram suggests little chance of hepatotoxicity, N-acetylcysteine can be discontinued.

N-acetylcysteine can be administered orally: a loading dose of 140 mg/kg body weight is followed by 70 mg/kg every 4 hours for an additional 17 doses. However, N-acetylcysteine smells and tastes terrible, and nausea and vomiting often limit oral administration. Diluting N-acetylcysteine with cola or juice or delivering it via a feeding tube may be helpful. An intravenous preparation has been available in Europe for some years and has recently become available in the USA. An infusion of 150 mg/kg (loading dose) is given over 15 minutes, followed by 50 mg/kg infusion over 4 hours and the last 100 mg/kg is infused over the remaining 16 hours.

The development of progressive liver failure with encephalopathy mandates the transfer of the patient to a liver transplant center. Indications for liver transplant are:

- PT greater than 100 seconds and serum creatinine greater than 300 µmol/L (3.4 mg/dL) in patients with grade III or IV encephalopathy

  or

- arterial blood pH below 7.3 (irrespective of grade of encephalopathy).

Isoniazid is a mainstay of treatment for both active and latent tuberculosis. Two types of hepatotoxicity are recognized. The first, and by far most common, is a transient mild elevation in the aminotransferases that occurs within a few months of beginning therapy. This occurs in approximately 20% of patients and is asymptomatic. Isoniazid should be continued and the patient monitored for symptoms and worsening liver tests. Often the liver test abnormalities will resolve despite continuing isoniazid.

Clinically evident isoniazid hepatitis, the second and much more serious form, is rare, occurring in fewer than 1% of treated patients. Fatal reactions are very rare (about 0.023%). About half of patients with clinical isoniazid hepatitis will develop symptoms within a few months of starting the drug, although presentations after as long as

TABLE 4.2

Risk factors for severe isoniazid hepatotoxicity

- Patient < 5 years or > 35 years of age
- Alcoholism
- Pre-existing liver disease (viral hepatitis)
- Acquired immunodeficiency syndrome
- Concomitant use of rifampin (rifampicin) and/or pyrazinamide (both of which have been reported to cause liver injury)

12 months have been reported. The presentation is similar to acute viral hepatitis, so these infections should be excluded. Isoniazid should be stopped immediately and the patient observed closely. Ideally, an alternative tuberculosis regimen should be substituted after the hepatitis resolves; however, isoniazid may be restarted with intensive monitoring when symptoms resolve and the aminotransferases fall below twice the upper limit of normal.

At a minimum, patients who start taking isoniazid should be educated to recognize and report any symptoms suggestive of liver dysfunction. Patients with symptoms should be evaluated promptly and thoroughly. Guidelines for monitoring asymptomatic patients for hepatotoxicity vary. The US Centers for Disease Control recommend liver tests before treatment and then periodically during treatment only in patients at high risk for hepatotoxicity (Table 4.2). Others, reasoning that concomitant use of other drugs with hepatotoxic potential (rifampin [rifampicin] and pyrazinamide) is so common, recommend liver tests at regular intervals.

Key points – drug-induced liver disease

- Drug-induced liver disease is common and usually mild.
- Determining the temporal relationship between starting a drug and the development of symptoms and signs of liver disease is important.
- Discontinuation of offending agents usually results in prompt resolution of hepatic injury.
- Monitoring for hepatotoxicity may be appropriate for some medications, such as statins and isoniazid.

Key references

American Thoracic Society, Centers for Disease Control and Prevention, Infectious Diseases Society of America. Treatment of tuberculosis. *Am J Respir Crit Care Med* 2003; 167:603–65.

Chalasani N, Aljadhey H, Kesterson J et al. Patients with elevated liver enzymes are not at higher risk for statin hepatotoxity. *Gastroenterology* 2004;126:1293–1301.

Lee WM. Acute liver failure in the United States. *Semin Liver Dis* 2003;23:217–26.

O'Grady JG, Alexander GJ, Hayllar KM, Williams R. Early indicators of prognosis in fulminant hepatic failure. *Gastroenterology* 1989; 97:439–45.

Rumack BH, Matthew H. Acetaminophen poisoning and toxicity. *Pediatrics* 1975;55:871–6.

Three liver diseases are categorized as autoimmune in etiology:
- autoimmune hepatitis (AIH), which targets the hepatocyte
- primary biliary cirrhosis (PBC), which affects the microscopic bile ducts
- primary sclerosing cholangitis (PSC), which can involve any elements of the intrahepatic and extrahepatic biliary system.

AIH and PBC are predominantly autoimmune diseases, but the categorization is less clear-cut with PSC. The classic immunologic profiles associated with these conditions are shown in Table 5.1. Some diagnostic confusion can occur because of the existence of 'overlap syndromes' or histological progression from apparent AIH to either PBC or PSC.

Autoimmune hepatitis

AIH is a chronic inflammatory liver disease of at least 6 months' duration. The target cell for the immunologic response is the

TABLE 5.1

Immunologic profiles in autoimmune liver diseases

Antibody	AIH	PBC	PSC
Antinuclear	++	+	++
Anti-smooth-muscle	+++	–	–
Anti-LKM*	+++	–	–
Antimitochondrial	–	+++	–
Elevated IgG	+++	–	+
Elevated IgM	–	++	–

–, not found; +, ++ and +++ indicate relative levels of antibodies.
* Type 2 AIH.
AIH, autoimmune hepatitis; Ig, immunoglobulin; LKM, liver–kidney microsomal; PBC, primary biliary cirrhosis; PSC, primary sclerosing cholangitis.

hepatocyte, and the dominant effector cells are lymphocytes and plasma cells. Two types of AIH are defined by classic autoantibody profiles:

- type 1: anti-smooth-muscle antibodies with or without antinuclear factor
- type 2: anti-liver-kidney microsomal antibodies.

These antibodies are associated with hypergammaglobulinemia, with a dominant elevation in the immunoglobulin (Ig) G fraction in untreated disease. Histological verification and staging of the disease is mandatory. The classic finding on liver histology is portal inflammation, with plasma cells and lymphocytes spilling over into the lobule in a pattern called interface hepatitis (Figure 5.1). Fibrosis or cirrhosis may be established by the time of presentation or may develop during follow-up despite apparently adequate therapy.

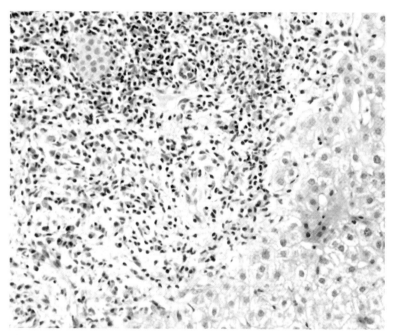

Figure 5.1 Interface hepatitis with 'spill-over' of inflammatory cells from the portal tract through the limiting plate into the liver parenchyma. This is the histological hallmark of untreated chronic autoimmune hepatitis. (Magnification × 200; picture courtesy of Dr A Knisley.)

Clinical features. There is a strong gender association, with 70% of cases occurring in women. The age at presentation has a bimodal distribution, with peaks during the second decade and the fourth and fifth decades.

AIH can present as an acute hepatitis-like illness, with jaundice and a laboratory profile showing hyperbilirubinemia and a marked elevation in serum aminotransferases (transaminases). A liver biopsy will show the characteristic features, with or without fibrosis or cirrhosis. Alternatively, patients may present with established cirrhosis in the absence of any previous episode of jaundice or other symptoms alerting to the presence of chronic hepatitis. These patients may present with liver failure or complications of portal hypertension. As with all causes of cirrhosis, there is a risk of hepatocellular carcinoma, but this risk is at the lower end of the spectrum in this condition.

Treatment. The standard treatment for AIH is immunosuppression with corticosteroids and azathioprine. Initial control is achieved with corticosteroids (e.g. prednisone, 30–60 mg/day). The dose is gradually reduced over 2–3 months to a target dose of 5–10 mg/day. Azathioprine is added as a steroid-sparing strategy and can be effective in maintaining remission, even after complete withdrawal of corticosteroids. Newer immunosuppressive drugs, such as mycophenolate and tacrolimus, are being used in refractory cases, but are not considered standard treatments for AIH.

The serum aminotransferases and IgG levels are used to monitor response to therapy. However, the intensity of necro-inflammatory activity may be understated by the serum aminotransferase levels, and repeat biopsy is recommended to confirm disease remission or if withdrawal of immunosuppressive therapy is being considered. Flares in disease activity occur in patients on stable long-term therapy and after reductions in drug dose. These flares are treated in a similar way to newly diagnosed disease.

Liver transplantation is an effective therapy for advanced disease. AIH recurs in up to 40% of cases but is generally easily controlled by inclusion of a higher dose of corticosteroids in the maintenance immunosuppression regimen.

Primary biliary cirrhosis

PBC is a progressive disease with an asymptomatic phase that may last for 15–20 years. The asymptomatic phase is being increasingly recognized, however, with the detection of increased alkaline phosphatase levels on routine blood tests. The diagnosis is effectively established by the detection of positive antimitochondrial antibodies (AMA), usually of the M2 subtype. The IgM fraction of the serum gammaglobulins is normally raised. The combination of elevated alkaline phosphatase, positive AMA and elevated IgM is now considered diagnostic of PBC and histological verification is no longer necessary. However, a liver biopsy may be of value in staging the severity of the disease.

The first symptoms are usually pruritus (itch) and lethargy (tiredness). The cause of the itch is unclear, but it responds in many cases to therapies that deplete bile salts (e.g. colestyramine). Antihistamines are not effective in this situation. The therapies used to treat the pruritus are listed in Table 5.2. The cause of the lethargy is also unclear, but there is increasing evidence to suggest that it is 'central' and secondary to changes within the brain. Hypothyroidism develops in up to 20% of patients with PBC, so it is important to screen regularly for this as a cause of the lethargy.

The development of jaundice indicates that the disease is entering the final stage, which lasts for 3–5 years. The prolonged cholestasis leads to cholesterol deposition in the skin (xanthomas and xanthelasma) and osteopenia or osteoporosis (Figure 5.2). At this stage, patients may also

TABLE 5.2

Treatments used for pruritus in primary biliary cirrhosis

- Colestyramine (cholestyramine)
- Ursodeoxycholic acid
- Rifampin (rifampicin)
- Naltrexone
- Ondansetron

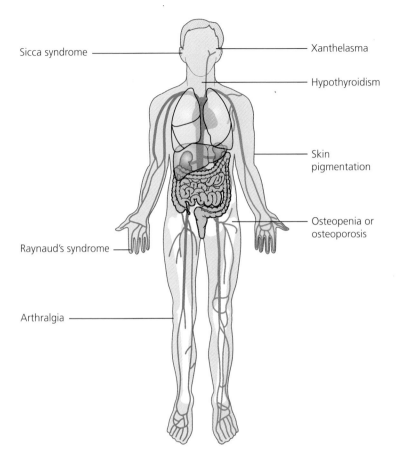

Sicca syndrome

Xanthelasma

Hypothyroidism

Skin pigmentation

Osteopenia or osteoporosis

Raynaud's syndrome

Arthralgia

Figure 5.2 Extrahepatic associations in primary biliary cirrhosis.

exhibit signs of portal hypertension, with ascites and esophageal or gastric varices. Encephalopathy is less common than in other causes of end-stage chronic liver disease.

There is no curative medical therapy for PBC. There is some evidence to support treatment with ursodeoxycholic acid (UDCA), as this improves the biochemical profile and possibly the histological appearance. There is, however, limited evidence that UDCA prolongs survival or delays the need for liver transplantation. A number of other immunosuppressive and antifibrotic therapies have failed to demonstrate sufficient benefit to gain widespread use.

45

Liver transplantation is still the only effective treatment for advanced PBC. The indications for transplantation are:

- serum bilirubin above 100–150 µmol/L (6–10 mg/dL)
- evidence of liver failure or severe portal hypertension at lower serum bilirubin levels
- severe intractable pruritus or lethargy
- severe osteoporosis
- complicating hepatocellular carcinoma.

The results of liver transplantation for PBC are excellent. There is evidence that PBC recurs in the transplanted liver, but this phenomenon appears to be of little clinical relevance in the first 10–15 years after transplantation.

Primary sclerosing cholangitis

PSC can affect all elements of the biliary system. Cholangiography classically shows diffuse stricturing and beading involving both the intrahepatic and extrahepatic bile ducts. In some cases, the extrahepatic bile ducts are spared, and confidence in making the diagnosis on radiological criteria is reduced. Liver histology may show the characteristic lesion of concentric fibrosis around the small bile ducts, termed 'onion-skin' fibrosis. The characteristic autoantibody is perinuclear antineutrophil cytoplasmic antibody (pANCA), but other autoantibodies may also be detected. Hypergammaglobulinemia occurs, with a predominant increase in the IgM fraction.

There is a strong association between PSC and inflammatory disease involving the large bowel – mainly ulcerative colitis but also Crohn's disease. About 75% of patients with PSC have inflammatory bowel disease and up to 7.5% of patients with ulcerative colitis have PSC. The diagnosis of PSC may be suggested by the detection of elevated cholestatic enzymes, particularly alkaline phosphatase, on routine screening of patients with inflammatory bowel disease. More advanced disease presents with jaundice and symptoms of biliary obstruction (dark urine, pale stools, itch) or low-grade cholangitis (fevers, sweats, feeling intermittently hot and cold).

The natural history of PSC is less predictable than that of PBC. Fluctuations in disease may:

- settle spontaneously
- respond to antibiotic therapy
- respond to treatment with UDCA
- improve after endoscopic dilation of a dominant stricture.

A rapid deterioration may indicate the development of a complicating cholangiocarcinoma. The risk of this malignant transformation is about 15% over the course of the disease. Screening for malignant transformation is not effective in detecting early disease, and progression to cholangiocarcinoma is generally regarded as a contraindication to liver transplantation.

UDCA, 10–15 mg/kg/day, is recommended. This ameliorates pruritus, improves the liver biochemistry and histology and may alter the natural history of the disease. Immunosuppressive and antifibrotic therapies have not proved effective. Liver transplantation is used widely for advanced disease. The indications for transplantation are less precise than they are in PBC, but persistent jaundice of more than 3 months' duration, in addition to evidence of liver failure or severe portal hypertension, are reasonable indications to proceed to liver transplantation. The fear of cholangiocarcinoma rendering an otherwise good transplant candidate unsuitable for transplantation has lowered the threshold for proceeding to transplantation in many centers. The results of liver transplantation are excellent in the absence of cholangiocarcinoma. PSC recurs in 8–15% of cases and is occasionally a cause of significant graft dysfunction.

Overlap syndromes

Diagnostic confusion may arise in some patients who manifest features of more than one autoimmune disease. Patients with early PBC may have florid interface hepatitis on liver biopsy, but this should not be confused with AIH. Other patients have features of AIH and a cholangiopathy and these are considered to have an 'overlap syndrome' or autoimmune cholangiopathy. These patients are managed as if they had both diseases (i.e. with corticosteroids and UDCA).

Key points – autoimmune liver diseases

- Autoimmune liver disease can target the hepatocyte or any element of the bile duct system.
- Autoimmune hepatitis (AIH) is potentially treatable if diagnosed before the development of cirrhosis.
- Primary biliary cirrhosis (PBC) is a slowly progressive disease, with a presymptomatic period of up to 20 years.
- Liver transplantation is an excellent treatment for end-stage AIH and PBC.
- Primary sclerosing cholangitis is strongly associated with ulcerative colitis and is unpredictable; late disease can be managed effectively with liver transplantation unless complicated by cholangiocarcinoma.

Key references

Durazzo M, Premoli A, Fagoonee S, Pellicano R. Overlap syndromes of autoimmune hepatitis: what is known so far. *Dig Dis Sci* 2003;48: 423–30.

Levy C, Lindor KD. Current management of primary biliary cirrhosis and primary sclerosing cholangitis. *J Hepatol* 2003;38: S24–37.

McFarlane IG. Autoimmune hepatitis: diagnostic criteria, subclassifications, and clinical features. *Clin Liver Dis* 2002:6: 317–33.

Poupon RE, Lindor KD, Cauch-Dudek K et al. Combined analysis of randomised controlled trials of ursodeoxycholic acid in primary biliary cirrhosis. *Gastroenterology* 1997;113:884–90.

Talwalkar JA, Lindor KD. Primary biliary cirrhosis. *Lancet* 2003:362; 53–61.

6 Metabolic liver diseases

Non-alcoholic fatty liver disease (NAFLD)

NAFLD is a group of disorders of diverse etiology (Table 6.1) and presents as a spectrum of disease ranging from apparently innocuous deposition of fat in the liver to cirrhosis with liver failure. Once thought to be uncommon and benign, NAFLD is now recognized as one of the most common forms of serious liver disease in Western populations. The growing prevalence of disorders associated with NAFLD (particularly diabetes, obesity and hyperlipidemia) suggests that fatty liver disease will be an important cause of morbidity and even mortality in the future. This discussion focuses on steatosis associated with insulin resistance.

Simple steatosis is the initial, and presumably most benign, type of NAFLD. Microscopically, fat droplets are seen in the hepatocytes and there is no or minimal inflammatory component. Simple steatosis is the most predictable form of fatty liver disease, occurring in many patients with diabetes and/or obesity. In the second, more advanced stage, an inflammatory response accompanies the fat. This lesion is termed non-alcoholic steatohepatitis (NASH). The liver cells balloon and are surrounded by inflammatory cells. Mallory bodies may be seen in the cytoplasm. The most advanced stages of NAFLD are marked by

TABLE 6.1

Common conditions associated with fatty liver

- Insulin resistance
  - diabetes
  - obesity
  - hyperlipidemia
- Starvation and rapid weight loss
- Parenteral nutrition
- Medications
  - glucocorticoids
  - methotrexate
  - amiodarone
  - antiretrovirals

49

deposition of collagen in the liver, resulting in progressive fibrosis and eventually the architectural distortion that signifies cirrhosis. These later two stages are unpredictable and develop from simple steatosis in a minority of patients.

Pathogenesis. The pathogenesis of NAFLD is incompletely understood. Insulin resistance plays an important role in the disease of the majority of patients with hepatic steatosis, namely those with obesity, diabetes and hyperlipidemia. Insulin resistance results in a complex cascade of events that increases triglyceride delivery to, and decreases triglyceride secretion from, the liver. The net result is accumulation of fat in the hepatocytes. How simple steatosis leads to inflammation and fibrosis is not known. A current theory suggests that mitochondrial fatty acid metabolism leads to the production of reactive oxygen species, which results in lipid peroxidation. Altered lipids are substrates for immune attack, which promotes the elaboration of cytokines from immune effector cells, leading to further cell injury. Peroxidized lipids and cytokines appear to promote activation of collagen-producing stellate cells, eventually resulting in cirrhosis.

Clinical presentation and diagnosis. Most patients with the early stages of NAFLD have few symptoms and are typically first identified by abnormal liver tests on routine screening. Hepatomegaly may be noted, but unless cirrhosis has developed with portal hypertension and/or liver failure, the examination is often unrevealing. The aminotransferases are usually mildly elevated, with alanine aminotransferase (ALT) typically higher than aspartate aminotransferase (AST) – an important characteristic. The ratio of the aminotransferases is helpful in excluding alcoholic liver injury – in ALD, AST is usually higher than ALT.

Because there is no specific laboratory test for NAFLD, most practitioners make a tentative diagnosis by excluding other causes of liver disease. Negative serology for hepatitis B and C rule out these chronic viral infections. Negative antinuclear and anti-smooth-muscle antibodies help rule out AIH. Inquiry regarding the use of prescribed and over-the-counter medications and nutritional supplements, particularly if there is a known temporal association between drug use and liver injury, helps to eliminate drug-induced injury. The possibility of drug-induced liver disease (see Chapter 4, Drug-induced liver disease) warrants attention, given that many patients take a variety of medications for disorders associated with NAFLD (diabetes, obesity and hyperlipidemia), and some of these medications have been reported to cause hepatic injury. Without a definitive method to quantify alcohol intake accurately, separating ALD from NAFLD remains problematic; histologically, they may be indistinguishable. The aminotransferase ratio – ALT higher than AST – and an accurate history from the patient and family members are helpful. However, the cautious physician will remember that obtaining an accurate alcohol history is quite difficult.

Imaging studies (ultrasonography and computed tomography) can detect significant hepatic steatosis. However, these studies cannot determine if inflammation or fibrosis accompanies the fat. There is currently no consensus on which patients require a liver biopsy to confirm the diagnosis of NAFLD. Many healthcare providers feel that in the appropriate patient (i.e. with obesity, diabetes and hyperlipidemia), in whom other disorders have been eliminated, the diagnosis of NAFLD is likely and a biopsy would be unlikely to alter treatment. It should be recognized, however, that the advanced forms of NAFLD cannot be reliably separated from simple fat without a biopsy. Thus, liver biopsy still plays an important role both in the ultimate diagnosis of the disorder and in determining prognosis.

The natural history of NAFLD is incompletely defined. Early descriptions of the disorder suggested that the course was essentially benign, whereas current evidence is less optimistic. Many patients have an uneventful course; however, some will advance to end-stage liver disease and are vulnerable to all the complications of cirrhosis. Older age and severe obesity are risks for advanced liver disease.

Treatment. Weight reduction is the mainstay of treatment for NAFLD. Patients should be strongly encouraged to lose weight slowly, as there is some evidence to suggest that rapid weight loss may provoke inflammation and even liver failure. Unfortunately, weight loss is extraordinarily difficult for most patients and success is often not achieved. However, the patient should be encouraged with the knowledge that weight loss is almost always associated with an improvement in liver tests and perhaps liver function. Careful control of diabetes and hyperlipidemia is recommended, although this may not affect the underlying liver disease. Currently no medications are universally accepted to alter the course of NAFLD. The insulin-sensitizing medications are logical choices. Promising results have been seen with thiazolidinediones (pioglitazone, rosiglitazone), vitamin E, metformin and gemfibrazole, but further controlled studies are required before recommending their use.

Hemochromatosis

Hemochromatosis is an inherited disorder of iron overload. Although common, it is underdiagnosed. It is now possible to test for the genetic markers associated with this disorder, and we hope that these tests will alter diagnostic acumen and lead to early discovery and treatment of patients with hemochromatosis.

Pathogenesis. The proximal intestine regulates iron balance.
- When there is a relative systemic deficiency of iron, absorption of iron from food is facilitated.
- When body stores are replete, absorption is downregulated and iron balance is maintained.
- There is no normal process for eliminating excessive body iron.

Genetic mutations associated with hemochromatosis result in altered regulation of iron absorption. Although the exact mechanism is not yet fully defined, the downregulation of iron absorption that normally accompanies the iron-replete state does not occur in patients with hemochromatosis. Rather, iron absorption continues and excessive stores are deposited in a variety of body tissues.

In hemochromatosis, unregulated iron absorption continues uninterrupted from birth. Critical tissue levels of iron (levels high enough to initiate injury) occur after more than 30 years, first in men and later in women (who are somewhat 'protected' while they lose iron during menstruation).

Excess iron appears to promote the generation of oxygen free radicals, which interact with lipid-rich membranes to form lipid peroxides. This results in membrane damage, cell death and promotion of fibrosis. After years of uncontrolled iron accumulation and injury, extensive fibrosis (cirrhosis) develops, resulting in organ dysfunction.

Clinical presentation. Most patients with hemochromatosis complain of fatigue and some will report arthralgia and loss of libido. Unfortunately, however, hemochromatosis has no specific symptoms and the disease is usually not suspected until significant, often irreversible, organ damage has occurred. Excessive iron is deposited in many organs and causes injury (Table 6.2). Age (older), gender (men), alcohol abuse, oral iron intake (supplements) and infection with hepatitis C may potentiate disease expression.

Diagnosis. The key to diagnosing hemochromatosis is to have a high index of suspicion. Unexplained cirrhosis or heart failure (particularly if diabetes is present) should raise concern. Often, abnormal iron studies are the only indications of the disease. Liver function tests (AST, ALT and alkaline phosphatase) are typically normal or only slightly elevated.

TABLE 6.2

Manifestations of hemochromatosis

Organ	Result
Liver	Cirrhosis Hepatocellular carcinoma
Heart	Pump failure* Arrhythmia*
Pancreas	Diabetes*
Skin	Increased pigmentation*
Pituitary	Hypogonadism
Joints	Arthritis – metacarpophalangeal joints

* Possibly reversible with treatment.

Liver functional parameters are non-specific and reflect the severity of liver dysfunction. Blood glucose levels may be elevated, reflecting destruction of pancreatic islets.

Transferrin saturation is a better diagnostic tool than ferritin concentration, which is often elevated in inflammatory conditions and non-hemochromatosis liver disorders. A transferrin saturation (serum iron divided by transferrin concentration) greater than 50% is suggestive of hemochromatosis. A ferritin concentration greater than twice the upper limit of normal deserves further investigation (Table 6.3).

The *HFE* gene plays an important, although incompletely defined, role in the regulation of iron absorption. Mutations in this gene are associated with hemochromatosis, and blood tests for the gene are commercially available. The most common mutation is cysteine to tyrosine at residue 282 (C282Y mutation) and is seen in most patients with the disease. Single copies of the mutation are relatively common in unselected populations (approximately 2%) but are much more common in some ethnic groups (approximately 10% of Irish). A histidine-to-aspartic-acid mutation at residue 63 (the H63D mutation) has also been described and appears to be more common but less severe than the C282Y mutation.

Patients who are homozygous for the C282Y mutation (C282Y/C282Y) are at greatest risk for significant iron overload

TABLE 6.3

Tests for hemochromatosis

Laboratory test	Hemochromatosis	Normal
Transferrin saturation (%)	> 50%	15–45
Ferritin (ng/dL)	> 600	< 300
Genetic markers	C282Y/C282Y	
Hepatic iron (mmol/g liver)	> 70	< 40
Hepatic iron index*	> 1.9	< 1.5

* The hepatic iron index is calculated by dividing the hepatic iron concentration by the patient's age.

and end-organ damage, whereas patients with one copy of each mutation (C282Y/H63D) are at less risk. Patients who are heterozygous for the C282Y mutation typically do not develop pathologic iron overload. The clinical significance of homozygosity for the H63D mutation (H63D/H63D) has been questioned – it may not predispose to pathologic iron overload. It is important to recognize that not all patients with hemochromatosis have typical mutations. Similarly, not all patients with typical mutations will develop pathologic iron overload – the penetration of the mutations is not yet understood.

Liver biopsy can be helpful in diagnosing hemochromatosis, as iron can be directly determined in a liver biopsy sample by chemical methods. A hepatic iron index, calculated from the hepatic iron concentration and the patient's age, is regarded as the gold standard for the diagnosis of the disorder. Iron stains show excessive parenchymal deposition of iron, but this method is, at best, semi-quantitative. The hepatology community is divided on the need to perform a liver biopsy to confirm the diagnosis in patients suspected of having hemochromatosis on the basis of serum iron studies and/or genetic tests. In general, it is recommended that patients with abnormal liver blood tests or other signs of liver disease undergo liver biopsy to confirm the diagnosis and determine the presence and severity of fibrosis.

Treatment. Reduction of systemic iron overload is the foundation of management for hemochromatosis. Therapeutic phlebotomy (Table 6.4), involving removal of one unit of blood (approximately 500 mL) approximately once a week, is necessary until the patient is iron-deficient (ferritin < 50 ng/dL). Once iron deficiency is achieved, the frequency of phlebotomy can be reduced to once every 2–4 months to maintain a low ferritin concentration. Alcohol consumption and iron supplements should be avoided, as should vitamin C supplements, as vitamin C facilitates iron absorption. Some physicians recommend oral antioxidants (vitamin E in particular), to help ameliorate iron-induced oxidation.

Hepatocellular carcinoma. Patients with hemochromatosis, particularly men with fibrotic disease, are at significant risk for HCC.

55

TABLE 6.4

Phlebotomy protocol for the management of hemochromatosis

- Stop all iron supplements and limit alcohol intake
- Begin phlebotomy:
  - remove one unit of blood (approximately 500 mL) every week*
  - check hematocrit before each phlebotomy; proceed if > 35%
  - continue until ferritin < 50 ng/dL (usually 1 year!)
- Once ferritin < 50 ng/dL, reduce phlebotomies to every 2–4 months
- Adjust phlebotomy schedule to keep ferritin < 50ng/dL; continue for life

* Some blood banks accept blood from patients with hemochromatosis.

It is reasonable to screen all patients with cirrhosis periodically (e.g. every 6–12 months) with serum alpha fetoprotein (AFP) determination and ultrasound imaging of the liver.

Screening for hemochromatosis. Because hemochromatosis is an easily treatable autosomal dominant disorder but has potentially devastating consequences, screening for the disorder is appealing. Early diagnosis allows for reduction of iron overload before injury occurs. Close relatives of patients identified with hemochromatosis should be screened by measuring transferrin saturation and genetic markers.

There is currently no consensus on screening the general population for hemochromatosis, although it appears logical to screen populations with the highest prevalence of the disease (those of northern European decent). A single measurement of transferrin saturation at 30 years of age in men and 40 years of age in women may be appropriate in these groups.

Wilson's disease

Wilson's disease is an autosomal recessive disorder of copper homeostasis. The defect involves mutation in the gene that codes for a canalicular copper 'pump', leading to impaired excretion of copper into bile. Excessive accumulation of copper in the liver, brain and other tissues leads to organ dysfunction (Table 6.5). The disorder is uncommon (1 in 30 000) and affects all races.

Symptoms and signs of Wilson's disease typically develop in older children and young adults, although in a few patients the disease is not discovered until the fifth or sixth decade. Younger patients usually present with hepatic dysfunction, whereas neuropsychiatric manifestations dominate the presentation of older patients.

The diagnosis of Wilson's disease rests on maintaining a high degree of suspicion for the disorder. All young patients with abnormal liver tests, signs of liver disease or any unexplained neuropsychiatric disorder deserve investigation. Serum ceruloplasmin is low in 95% of patients with Wilson's disease. Definitive diagnosis rests on documenting excessive hepatic copper by liver biopsy (Table 6.6).

The mainstay of treatment involves chelation of copper, allowing for urinary excretion. Penicillamine is the drug of choice, and trientine is used for the 30% of patients who are intolerant of penicillamine. Oral zinc appears to interfere with copper absorption by the small bowel and has been used as an adjunct to chelation therapy.

TABLE 6.5

Clinical manifestations of copper deposition in Wilson's disease

Organ	Clinical manifestations of copper deposition
Liver	Asymptomatic elevation of liver function tests Acute/chronic hepatitis Fulminant hepatic failure Cirrhosis
Brain	Tremor Ataxia Personality change/depression
Eye	Kayser–Fleischer rings
Red blood cells	Hemolysis
Kidney	Proximal renal tubular acidosis Hypouricemia

TABLE 6.6

Diagnostic tests for Wilson's disease

Test	Wilson's disease	Normal
Ceruloplasmin concentration	< 20 mg/dL	20–45 mg/dL
24-hour urinary copper excretion	> 100 µg	< 35 µg
Hepatic copper concentration	> 250 µg/g liver	< 50 µg/g liver

α_1 antitrypsin deficiency (ATD)

ATD is a well-known cause of chronic lung disease. It is also associated with liver disease in children and adults. Although ATD is not rare (it affects approximately 1 in 1800 births), only a small percentage of patients with ATD will develop liver disease. The hepatic manifestations of ATD are listed in Table 6.7. Low serum levels of α_1 antitrypsin, a consistent protease inhibitor phenotype (i.e. protease inhibitor homozygous for the Z mutation; PiZZ) and a liver biopsy that reveals PAS-staining granules in hepatocytes confirm the diagnosis. There is no specific treatment for ATD liver disease. Transplant is an option for patients with advanced liver disease.

TABLE 6.7

Hepatic manifestations of α_1 antitrypsin deficiency

Children	Adults
• Coagulopathy	• Chronic hepatitis
• Protracted jaundice	• Cirrhosis
• Neonatal hepatitis	• Hepatocellular carcinoma

Key points – metabolic liver diseases

- Non-alcoholic fatty liver disease (NAFLD) is a common liver disorder, most often seen in obese or diabetic patients.
- NAFLD is a spectrum of conditions from simple steatosis to cirrhosis with liver failure.
- When associated with obesity, NAFLD is best treated with weight loss.
- Hemochromatosis is easily treatable but underdiagnosed.
- It is reasonable to screen patients at risk of hemochromatosis by measuring the transferrin saturation in early middle age.

Key references

Angulo P. Nonalcoholic fatty liver disease. *N Engl J Med* 2002;346:1221–31.

Brandhagen DJ, FairbanksVF, Baldus W. Recognition and management of hereditary hemochromatosis. *Am Fam Physician* 2002;65:853–60.

Bulaj ZJ, Griffin LM, Jorde LB et al. Clinical and biochemical abnormalities in people heterozygous for hemochromatosis. *N Engl J Med* 1996;335:1799.

Clark JM, Brancati FL, Diehl AM. Nonalcoholic fatty liver disease. *Gastroenterology* 2002;122:1649–57.

Cuthbert J. Wilson's disease: update of a systemic disorder with protean manifestations. *Gastroenterol Clin North Am* 1998;27:655–81.

Day CP. Non-alcoholic steatohepatitis (NASH): where are we now and where are we going? *Gut* 2002;50:585–8.

Gochhee PA, Powell LW. What's new in hemochromatosis. *Curr Opin Hematol* 2001;8:98–104.

Loudianos G, Gitlin J. Wilson's disease. *Semin Liver Dis* 2000;20:353–64.

McCarthy GM, McCarthy CJ, Kenny D et al. Hereditary hemochromatosis: a common, often unrecognized genetic disorder. *Cleve Clin J Med* 2002;69:224–37.

Perlmutter DH. Alpha-1-antitrypsin deficiency. *Semin Liver Disease* 1998;18:217–25.

Philpott CC. Molecular aspects of iron absorption: insights into the role of HFE in hemochromatosis. *Hepatology* 2002;35:993–1001.

Saadeh S, Younossi ZM, Remer EM et al. The utility of radiological imaging in nonalcoholic fatty liver disease. *Gasteroenterology* 2002;123:745–50.

Steinberg KK, Cogswell ME, Chang JC et al. Prevalance of C282Y and H63D mutations in the hemochromatosis (HFE) gene in the United States. *JAMA* 2001;285:2216–22.

Chronic infection with the hepatitis B (HBV) or C (HCV) virus is the most common cause of chronic liver disease worldwide (Table 7.1). There are an estimated 300 million hepatitis B carriers worldwide and the prevalence of hepatitis B ranges from 0.1 to 20%. The prevalence of hepatitis C also varies geographically and ranges from 0.5 to 15%. Hepatitis is considered chronic when the infection is present for more than 6 months.

Hepatitis B

The prevalence of hepatitis B infection varies worldwide; the highest rates are seen in Asia. The risk factors for acquisition of the virus are discussed in Chapter 1, Investigating liver disease (page 14).

Chronic hepatitis B is evaluated on the basis of serological profiles, liver function tests and, in some cases, liver histology. A number of patterns of disease are recognized:

- tolerant phase – the virus is replicating actively but there is no evidence of liver damage
- immune clearance phase – immune recognition results in attempts to control viral replication and may cause a clinically recognizable episode of hepatitis (this process can lead to clearance of the virus or to downregulation of viral replication without clearance of the virus)
- persistent replication with evidence of ongoing hepatitis
- intermittent flares in viral replication, which may trigger episodes of hepatitis
- established cirrhosis, with or without evidence of ongoing viral replication.

The serological evaluation of chronic hepatitis B can appear complex (Table 7.2). It utilizes two viral proteins – the 'surface' and 'e' antigens (HBsAg and HBeAg) – and their associated antibodies, in addition to hepatitis B DNA. HBsAg is present in all cases of chronic infection. The HBeAg/'e' antibody (HBeAb) status was previously used to determine whether individuals had active viral replication but,

TABLE 7.1

Comparison of hepatitis B and hepatitis C viruses

	Hepatitis B virus	Hepatitis C virus
Virus type	DNA	RNA
Prevalence – West	0.1–2%	0.5–1%
– highest	20% China	15% Africa
Worldwide burden	300 million	150 million
Vertical transmission	90%	5%
Sexual transmission	High	Low
Blood-product transmission	Low	Low since 1990–91
Vaccine available	Yes	No
Response to therapy	40–60%	50–85%*
Time to cirrhosis	≥ 5 years	25–30 years
Risk of cirrhosis	20%	25%
Recurrence after liver transplantation	15–20%	99%

* Depending on genotype.

TABLE 7.2

Serological evaluation of hepatitis B

HBsAg	HBsAb	HBeAg	HBeAb	HBV DNA	Status
–	+	–	+	–	Immune
+	–	+	–	+	Replicator
+	–	–	+	–	Non-replicator
+	–	–	+ or –	+	Pre-core mutant
+	–	–	–	–	Seroconverting

+, positive status; –, negative status; HBsAg/Ab, hepatitis B 'surface' antigen/antibody; HBeAg/Ab, hepatitis B 'e' antigen/antibody; HBV, hepatitis B virus.

although it remains a reasonable screening test, determination of the replication status by measuring HBV DNA levels in blood is now considered more accurate.

Pre-core mutants of the HBV do not express HBeAg, and infected individuals may not have HBeAb, unless they were previously infected with the wild-type virus. In these cases, the viral replication status can only be determined by HBV DNA assay. Seroconversion from HBeAg to HBeAb may cause hepatitis-like symptoms; patients come to clinical attention during this process. Such symptoms can also manifest when both HBeAg and HBeAb are negative. These patients have low HBV DNA levels and will later express HBeAb.

Natural history. Chronic hepatitis develops in 90% of infants and in 5% of adults acquiring the infection. The spectrum of liver disease associated with chronic hepatitis B includes:
- minimal change
- active inflammation with interface hepatitis
- fibrosis
- cirrhosis
- hepatocellular carcinoma (HCC) (usually, but not always, with associated cirrhosis).

Many patients with chronic hepatitis do not develop significant liver disease during their lifetime. The risk of progression to cirrhosis is about 20% over 5 years, and is greater in males than females. Once cirrhosis develops, 85% of patients remain stable for a further 5 years, but the risk of developing symptoms of liver failure increases significantly thereafter. The risk of developing HCC once cirrhosis has developed is 1–2% per year.

Treatment. There are two main approaches to the treatment of hepatitis B. Interferon clears the virus in about 40% of cases by increasing immune responsiveness to the virus. The standard dose is 9–10 million units given as a subcutaneous injection three times a week for 4–6 months. Alternatively, 5–6 million units can be administered daily. More recently, peginterferon has been used for the treatment of HBV infection. The potential side effects are significant (Table 7.3).

TABLE 7.3

Side effects of interferon therapy

- Flu-like symptoms on initiation
- Fatigue
- Anorexia and weight loss
- Alopecia
- Bone-marrow suppression
- Thyroid dysfunction
- Flares of latent autoimmunity
- Depression

Lamivudine and adefovir are nucleoside and nucleotide analogs, respectively, that reliably reduce viral replication and lead to seroconversion to HBeAb in 30–60% of cases with treatment regimens of 3 years or longer. Lamivudine is extremely well tolerated, but resistance to the drug emerges in a high proportion of cases. Adefovir, a newer drug, is slower acting but is ultimately more potent and has a very low resistance rate (about 2% at 1 year). The toxicity profile with extended use is less clearly understood than that for lamivudine.

Newer agents like tenofovir, entecavir and telbivudine are emerging, and it is possible that combination therapy will become the therapeutic approach of choice in the future.

Lamivudine or adefovir are preferred to interferon in patients with Child's B or C cirrhosis (see Table 12.6, page 100), as interferon carries a significant risk of triggering decompensation of the liver disease. They are also preferred in patients with high HBV DNA levels and when there are contraindications to interferon therapy (e.g. history of depression, thrombocytopenia, coexisting autoimmune disease). In other patients, the choice of therapy may depend on patient preference between a 'short sharp regimen' and a more protracted therapy but with significantly fewer side effects.

Liver transplantation is indicated for patients developing liver failure and those found to have small HCCs (typically 1–3 nodules with diameters not exceeding 5 cm on radiological evaluation). Liver decompensation associated with active viral replication has the potential to improve dramatically with lamivudine or adefovir, and patients apparently in need of liver transplantation can recover and defer the need for transplantation for many years. The overall burden of hepatitis B on transplant resources is therefore decreasing.

Passive immunoprophylaxis using hepatitis B immunoglobulin, possibly in combination with adefovir or lamivudine, is successful in preventing re-infection of the liver in over 80% of cases when the HBV DNA is negative at the time of liver transplantation. In the absence of re-infection, the results of liver transplantation for hepatitis B are comparable to those for the other patient subgroups.

Hepatitis D (delta) virus is an incomplete virus that can exist only in association with hepatitis B infection. It can be acquired with the hepatitis B or can be superimposed on established disease. It seems to lead to more aggressive liver disease, even though, paradoxically, it suppresses the replication of HBV. The incidence of hepatitis D appears to be decreasing. Currently, there are no good treatments.

Hepatitis C

Hepatitis C virus is an RNA virus. The recognized means of acquisition involves contact with blood, and the virus was commonly transmitted via blood products before the introduction of screening for hepatitis C in 1990–91. Intravenous drug use was associated with an infection rate of approximately 70%, and tattooing has resulted in infection with hepatitis C in up to 30% of cases. Sexual and vertical transmission are possible but unusual. The mode of acquisition in areas of high prevalence is unclear. The prevalence of hepatitis C varies geographically and ranges from 0.5–1% in most Western countries to over 15% in parts of Africa.

The serological assessment of hepatitis C includes:
- antibody to HCV as the initial screening test
- qualitative polymerase chain reaction (PCR) for HCV RNA as a screen for persistent infection
- quantitative PCR for HCV RNA as a guide to response to therapy
- HCV genotype.

There are four main genotypes of HCV.

- Genotype 1 is particularly prevalent in Western countries and in intravenous drug users.
- Genotypes 2 and 3 are most common in Northern Europe.
- Genotype 4 is most frequently encountered in Egypt.

The genotype is relevant when assessing the likely response to therapy and in determining the duration of therapy. Hepatitis C is also associated with a phenomenon called quasi-species, which denotes the presence of many strains of the virus within an individual patient.

Natural history. The acute infection is rarely clinically identified and, in most cases, the likely timing of infection can only be determined from an assessment of the risk factors for acquisition of the virus. About 85% of those infected become chronic carriers. Individuals are considered to have spontaneously cleared the virus if tests for HCV RNA are negative on three occasions over a period of at least 2 years.

Infected individuals express a range of liver disease, ranging from mild hepatitis to cirrhosis. The risk of progressing to cirrhosis is 25–30% over a period of up to 30 years. Alcohol consumption accelerates progression to cirrhosis by up to 10 years. Patients over 40 years of age also have more aggressive disease. Once cirrhosis develops, the superimposed risk of developing HCC is in the order of 1–2% per patient-year.

Once HCV antibodies have been detected, the patient should be screened for HCV RNA (Figure 7.1). Most patients with viremia should have a liver biopsy, even if the liver function profile is entirely in the normal range. The rationale for this is that serum aminotransferases (transaminases) regularly underestimate the intensity of the necro-inflammatory process and there is no reliable alternative way of assessing fibrosis. A liver biopsy may not be indicated if the HCV is genotype 2 or 3 and it is considered that the high response rate to therapy justifies treatment in the absence of significant liver injury. More commonly, and certainly for genotypes 1 and 4, antiviral therapy is directed at patients with interface hepatitis or significant fibrosis. Histological re-evaluation is recommended after 3–5 years in patients who do not meet criteria for antiviral therapy when initially assessed.

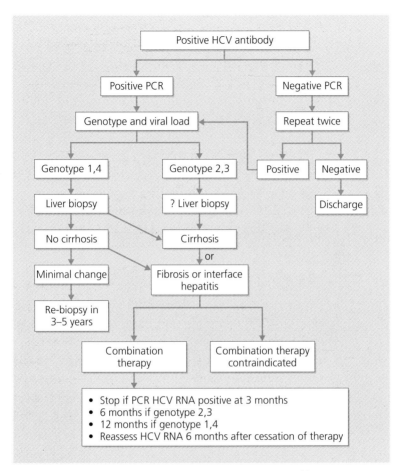

Figure 7.1 Algorithm for the assessment and treatment of hepatitis C. HCV, hepatitis C virus; PCR, polymerase chain reaction.

Treatment. The objective of therapy is to get a sustained virological response, which is defined as persistent absence of viremia (qualitative PCR for HCV RNA) more than 6 months after cessation of therapy. The best results have been obtained with the combination of peginterferon and ribavirin, so this has largely replaced older regimens with standard interferon (which was used in doses of 3–5 million units three times per week). The precise dosing regimen for peginterferon, which is given once weekly, depends on which of the proprietary preparations is used and the patient's weight. Ribavirin is given orally

67

at a dose of 1.0–1.2 g daily, but the dose may need to be modified if anemia develops.

Unresponsive patients can usually be identified by persistent viremia after 3 months' treatment, so therapy is discontinued in such patients at that time. Estimation of quantitative viral load may identify non-responders within the first month of therapy. In responders, treatment is continued for 6 months for genotypes 2 and 3, and for 12 months for genotypes 1 and 4. The overall response rates for patients without cirrhosis are 50–55% for genotypes 1 and 4 and 80–85% for genotypes 2 and 3. Response rates are lower in patients with cirrhosis, at around 30%. Characteristics that influence the response to therapy are summarized in Table 7.4.

Liver transplantation. Liver disease associated with hepatitis C is now the most common indication for liver transplantation in most countries. Unlike hepatitis B, the burden of hepatitis C on transplant resources is increasing and is not expected to peak for another 5–10 years. The indications for liver transplantation are the same as for hepatitis B. However, unlike hepatitis B, re-infection of the graft is almost inevitable as no immunoprophylaxis is currently available, although a proportion of patients who are HCV RNA negative at the time of transplantation following antiviral therapy do not develop recurrent infection. However, the majority of liver transplant candidates cannot tolerate antiviral therapy.

TABLE 7.4

Factors increasing response to therapy for hepatitis C

- Female
- Age < 40 years
- Abstinence from alcohol
- Genotypes 2 and 3
- Low viral load
- Absence of cirrhosis
- HIV seronegative

HIV, human immunodeficiency virus.

> **Key points – chronic viral hepatitis**
>
> - Hepatitis B and C are the most common causes of chronic liver disease and hepatocellular carcinoma worldwide.
> - Hepatitis B is preventable with vaccination and is treatable in 40–60% of cases.
> - There is no vaccine for hepatitis C, but it is treatable in 50–85% of cases (depending on genotype).
> - Liver transplantation is required for end-stage chronic liver disease and small hepatocellular carcinoma.
> - Hepatitis C almost invariably recurs after liver transplantation and is problematic.

A significant minority (20–30%) are at risk of accelerated disease, with cirrhosis developing as early as 3–5 years after transplantation. As a result, the survival rate for hepatitis C is lower than for other indications 8 years and more after liver transplantation. A number of risk factors for accelerated disease have been identified (Table 7.5). Treatment of recurrent disease with combination therapy is problematic because of enhanced drug toxicity.

TABLE 7.5

Factors associated with aggressive hepatitis C recurrence after liver transplantation

- Older male recipients
- High viral load before transplant
- Probably genotype 1
- Donor age > 50 years
- Steatotic grafts
- Multiple rejection episodes
- Intensity of immunosuppression

Key references

Alberti A, Benvegnu L. Management of hepatitis C. *J Hepatol* 2003:38(suppl 1):S104–118.

Conjeevaram HS, Lok As-F. Management of chronic hepatitis B. *J Hepatol* 2003:38(suppl 1);S90–103.

Hoofnagle J. Course and outcome of hepatitis C. *Hepatology* 2002;36:S21–9.

Cirrhosis is the end result of long-standing injuries to the liver of diverse etiology. Some patients will develop complications of cirrhosis, such as ascites, portal hypertensive bleeding and/or hepatic encephalopathy. These complications may be devastating and portend a poor prognosis.

Ascites

Ascites is the most common complication of cirrhosis and usually heralds a progressive downhill course. Approximately 50% of patients with ascites from cirrhosis will have died after 2 years. Although this chapter deals with ascites caused by cirrhosis, it should be remembered that cirrhosis is not the only cause of fluid accumulation in the abdomen (Table 8.1).

Evaluation. Most patients with cirrhosis will report developing abdominal distension as ascites develops. The patient should be questioned about history or risk factors for liver disease. A history of congestive heart failure, malignancy, pancreatic disease or trauma should be sought. Examination usually reveals a protuberant abdomen with shifting dullness and a fluid thrill. Other stigmata of liver disease (palmar erythema, spider nevi, telangiectasia, gynecomastia, etc.) are

TABLE 8.1

Etiology of ascites

- Liver disease/cirrhosis
- Malignancy
- Heart failure
- Infection (tuberculosis)
- Pancreatitis
- Lymphatic disruption

TABLE 8.2

Laboratory investigation of ascites

Investigation	Suggestive of
Appearance of ascites	
• Clear/yellow	Cirrhosis, congestive heart failure
• Bloody	Trauma, malignancy
• Milky	Lymphatic disruption
• Cloudy	Infection
SAAG	
• ≥ 1.1 g/dL	Portal hypertension (cirrhosis)
• < 1.1 g/dL	Malignancy
> 250 PMN/mL	Infection
Positive culture	Infection
Amylase	Pancreatitis
Triglycerides	Malignancy Disruption of thoracic duct

SAAG, serum–ascites albumin gradient (difference between serum albumin and ascites albumin concentrations); PMN, polymorphonuclear leukocytes.

usually present. Most patients have peripheral edema. Blood tests usually document evidence of liver dysfunction.

Diagnostic paracentesis is mandatory for all patients with new ascites (Table 8.2). Fluid obtained during paracentesis should be sent for measurement of albumin levels, cell count, cytology and culture (ascites should be inoculated into blood culture bottles at the bedside for optimal yield). A peripheral albumin level should be determined. The calculation of the serum–ascites albumin gradient (SAAG) has proved useful for distinguishing ascites associated with portal hypertension from other causes, and is 97% accurate. The SAAG is calculated by subtracting the ascites albumin level from the serum albumin level. If the difference is greater than or equal to 1.1 g/dL, the ascites is a consequence of portal hypertension. Amylase and triglyceride levels may be determined to evaluate ascites due to pancreatic disease or lymphatic disruption, respectively.

Treatment of the underlying liver disease is the optimal treatment of ascites (Table 8.3) but, unfortunately, may not be a practical option. All patients with ascites should restrict their dietary sodium intake to less than 2 g per day. (More severe restrictions are impracticable and may hinder general nutrition.) Fluid restriction is reserved for those patients with significant hyponatremia. Diuretics offer relief to many patients. Spironolactone, 100–200 mg daily, combined with furosemide, 40 mg daily, is an effective starting oral regimen. Typical maximum daily doses of spironolactone and furosemide are 400 mg and 160 mg, respectively. Renal function and electrolytes should be monitored frequently and the diuretics adjusted as needed. Rapid diuresis with intravenous diuretics often results in azotemia and electrolyte abnormalities, and should be undertaken with caution.

Large-volume paracentesis (LVP), or the removal of several liters of ascites, is enjoying a resurgence among hepatologists. Although once frowned upon, LVP has been shown by recent studies to be a safe and effective technique for the rapid treatment of ascites. Most practitioners remove up to 5 liters of fluid at a time, although some perform total paracentesis (removing all ascites at one tap) without ill effects. Diuretics should be discontinued a few days before LVP. Many authors recommend the intravenous infusion of albumin after LVP to prevent the systemic hyponatremia and circulatory dysfunction that can follow paracentesis; however, the clinical consequences of these abnormalities are unclear. Most practitioners reserve albumin infusion for patients without peripheral edema.

TABLE 8.3

Treatment of ascites

- Salt restriction
- Diuretics: spironolactone, furosemide
- Large-volume paracentesis
- Liver transplantation
- Transjugular intrahepatic portosystemic shunt (TIPS)

Transjugular intrahepatic portosystemic shunts (TIPS) may help patients with ascites refractory to other treatments. TIPS is a radiologic procedure in which an expandable metallic stent is tunneled through the hepatic parenchyma to connect the hypertensive portal vasculature to the low-pressure hepatic vein. TIPS is available in many hepatology referral centers. Peritoneovenous shunting has been largely abandoned.

Patients with refractory ascites should be considered for liver transplantation, provided they are otherwise good candidates (see Chapter 12, Liver transplantation).

Spontaneous bacterial peritonitis (SBP) should be suspected in a patient with ascites who is not doing well. The clinical findings associated with SBP may be subtle: fever and abdominal pain or tenderness are not common. Vague changes in mental status, electrolyte abnormalities or renal insufficiency may be the only signs and should prompt a diagnostic paracentesis. An ascitic neutrophil count above 250 cells/mm^3 suggests infection and mandates immediate antibiotic treatment, before cultures are available. A third-generation cephalosporin or ampicillin/sulbactam offers good empiric coverage for typical organisms. Aminoglycosides should be avoided.

Portal hypertensive bleeding

Esophagogastric varices are present in approximately 50% of patients with cirrhosis. Not all patients with varices will bleed, but those who do have a poor prognosis. Despite significant advances in treatment of patients who bleed, mortality remains extraordinarily high. Thus, preventing the first episode of bleeding (primary prevention) is essential for patients at risk.

Primary prevention. Patients with cirrhosis should be screened for varices by endoscopy. If varices of significant size are identified, prophylactic treatment should be started (Table 8.4). The mainstays of prophylactic treatment are non-selective beta-blockers: propranolol (starting dose 20 mg twice daily) or nadolol (40 mg daily) reduce the incidence of bleeding for patients with medium or large esophageal varices. The dosages are increased until the patient's heart rate is 50–60 beats per minute. Endoscopic band ligation may benefit patients

TABLE 8.4

Primary prevention of variceal bleeding

- Endoscopy screening of all cirrhotic patients
- Start non-selective beta-blockers in patients with high-risk varices:
  - nadolol 40 mg daily or
  - propranolol 20 mg twice daily
  - titrate dose to keep heart rate at 50–60 beats per min
- Consider band ligation for those with large varices who cannot tolerate beta-blockers

who cannot tolerate beta-blockers. Additional research is required before prophylaxis with nitrates can be recommended, and sclerotherapy is not recommended.

Active bleeding. Variceal bleeding is rarely subtle and should be suspected in any patient with gastrointestinal bleeding and a history or evidence of chronic liver disease. The patient often presents in extremis, hypotensive with hematemesis and melena. Resuscitation is the first step in treatment (Table 8.5). Crystalloids usually suffice to stabilize the patient initially, and blood is given to keep the hematocrit in a safe range. Overtransfusion (hematocrit above 30%) may precipitate further bleeding. Short-term antibiotic prophylaxis with norfloxacin has been shown to reduce the risk of infections that commonly follow variceal bleeding, and improves mortality. Prompt endoscopy will enable identification of varices and the opportunity to control active bleeding. Several techniques are available. In endoscopic variceal ligation (EVL), small rubber bands are used to ligate varices. EVL usually controls active bleeding with few complications. In endoscopic sclerotherapy (ES), a thin needle is advanced through the endoscope into the varix, and one of several available irritant sclerosants is injected into the varix. Like EVL, ES is effective in controlling bleeding. ES is often easier to perform in patients who are actively bleeding, but is associated with more complications than EVL.

Both EVL and ES help to prevent further episodes of bleeding (secondary prevention). After the first episode of bleeding, patients undergo EVL or ES on several occasions to obliterate the varices fully; typically, 3–5 sessions are needed.

Much attention had been devoted to the use of pharmacological agents for the control of acute variceal bleeding. Vasopressin in combination with intravenous nitroglycerin (glyceryl trinitrate) is effective in controlling variceal bleeding, but its many side effects have limited its use. Somatostatin and terlipressin control bleeding in approximately 75% of patients, but neither drug is available in the USA. Octreotide, a long-acting analog of somatostatin, has become the agent of choice in the USA, although available evidence regarding efficacy is controversial. The role of octreotide is undefined and it is best regarded as an adjunct to endoscopic techniques.

Transjugular intrahepatic portosystemic shunts (see Figure 2.2) or surgical portal decompressive shunts have a role in patients who have not responded to less dramatic interventions. Balloon tamponade is

TABLE 8.5

Treatment of active variceal bleeding

- Rapid resuscitation
- Blood transfusion to keep hematocrit at 25–30%
- Norfloxacin, 400 mg twice daily for 7 days
- Pharmacological agents (use depending on local availability):
  - somatostatin
  - terlipressin
  - octreotide
  - vasopressin/nitroglycerin
- Prompt endoscopy with EVL or ES to control bleeding
- Follow-up EVL/ES to obliterate varices
- TIPS/surgical shunt/balloon tamponade as rescue techniques

ES, endoscopic sclerotherapy; EVL, endoscopic variceal ligation; TIPS, transjugular intrahepatic portosystemic shunt.

effective in controlling bleeding, but an alarming list of associated complications limits its use, and it is currently regarded as a technique of last resort.

Hepatic encephalopathy

Hepatic encephalopathy encompasses a spectrum of neuropsychiatric abnormalities in patients with established liver disease in the absence of other metabolic or structural brain abnormalities. The pathogenesis of the disorder is not fully understood and is an area of active investigation and often heated debate. It is likely that gut-derived ammonia plays some role in the disorder, and theories of endogenous benzodiazepines, false neurotransmitters and brain edema have been postulated.

Hepatic encephalopathy can present with a wide range of neuropsychiatric impairment, from subtle alteration in mood, sleep and attention, to stupor and deep coma. Constipation, bleeding, a high-protein diet, electrolyte abnormalities, renal insufficiency and infection may precipitate the syndrome. There are no specific findings on physical examination. Asterixis is frequently elicited, but is not specific for hepatic encephalopathy. Venous ammonia levels are commonly determined in clinical practice, although there is very poor correlation between ammonia levels and clinical presentation. The diagnosis of hepatic encephalopathy rests upon eliminating other causes for changes in mental status (intoxication, narcosis, subdural hematoma, etc.) in a patient with advanced liver disease.

Treatment of hepatic encephalopathy (Table 8.6) should include correction of precipitating factors. Limiting protein in the diet is reasonable but should be recommended with some caution – many patients with cirrhosis are malnourished, and excessive protein restriction may prevent adequate nourishment. Benzodiazepines and narcotics should be avoided. Renal and electrolyte abnormalities are common in patients with cirrhosis who are taking diuretics, and should be corrected. Infections, particularly SBP, should be ruled out.

The mainstay of treatment is the non-absorbable disaccharide lactulose. Lactulose induces catharsis and acidifies the bowel lumen, resulting in the reduction of absorbable neurotoxins (ammonia?).

TABLE 8.6

Prevention and treatment of hepatic encephalopathy

- Moderate protein restriction
- Correction of renal and electrolyte abnormalities
- Treat infection
- Discontinue any sedatives/narcotics
- Lactulose orally or by enema
- Consider neomycin if lactulose fails

Oral lactulose, 15–30 mL one to three times a day, is given to stable patients to produce two or three soft bowel movements per day. Profuse diarrhea may contribute to renal insufficiency and should be avoided. Patients who are acutely encephalopathic often benefit from aggressive dosing until bowel movements occur. Tap-water enemas containing lactulose are used for patients unable to take oral lactulose. If lactulose fails, patients may benefit from neomycin, 1 g four times daily, although long-term use of neomycin can result in ototoxicity and nephrotoxicity.

Key points – complications of cirrhosis

- Diagnostic paracentesis is mandatory in any patient with new ascites.
- Salt restriction and diuretics are effective in most patients with ascites. Repeated large-volume paracentesis and TIPS may be required for refractory cases.
- Patients with cirrhosis should be screened for varices. If these are present, prophylactic treatment with β-blockers is recommended.
- Acute variceal bleeding is best treated with endoscopic techniques; however, pharmacotherapy also has a limited role.
- Hepatic encephalopathy is a diagnosis of exclusion. Lactulose and correction of precipitating factors are the mainstays of treatment.

Key references

Abou-Assi S, Vlahcevic ZR. Hepatic encephalopathy. Metabolic consequence of cirrhosis often is reversible. *Postgrad Med* 2001;109: 52–65.

Ferenci P, Lockwood A, Mullen K et al. Hepatic encephalopathy – definition, nomenclature, diagnosis, and quantification: final report of the working party at the 11th World Congresses of Gastroenterology, Vienna, 1998. *Hepatology* 2002; 35:716–21.

Gow PJ, Chapman RW. Modern management of oesophageal varices. *Postgrad Med J* 2001;77:77–81.

Grace ND, Groszmann RJ, Garcia-Tsao G et al. Portal hypertension and variceal bleeding. An AASLD single topic symposium. *Hepatology* 1998;28:868–80.

Jensen DM. Endoscopic screening for varices in cirrhosis: findings, implications, and outcomes. *Gastroenterology* 2002;112: 1620–30.

Lockwood AH. Hepatic encephalopathy. *Neurol Clin* 2002;20:241–6.

Runyon BA. Management of adult patients with ascites caused by cirrhosis. *Hepatology* 1998;27: 264–72.

VA web document. Treatment of patients with cirrhosis and portal hypertension. Version 1 (October 2003). www.hepatitis.va.gov/vahep?page= tp03-03-02-01

Weissenborn K, Ennen JC, Schomerus H et al. Neuropsychological characterization of hepatic encephalopathy. *J Hepatol* 2001;34:768–73.

Benign liver tumors, cysts, infections and abscesses

The use of ultrasonography in the investigation of abdominal symptoms and abnormal liver function tests has greatly increased the detection of benign liver lesions (Table 9.1), although the lesions identified are often not relevant to the issue under investigation. Because the detection of focal lesions in the liver can precipitate considerable anxiety until they are characterized as benign, appropriate investigations are warranted and occasionally therapeutic intervention is indicated.

The typical investigation pathway after the initial detection is by computed tomography (CT) or magnetic resonance imaging. The key questions to be answered about the lesion are:

- is it solid, cystic or both?
- is it vascular or avascular?

TABLE 9.1

Benign focal liver lesions

Common causes
- Simple cysts
- Hemangioma
- Focal nodular hyperplasia
- Adenoma

Rare lesions
- Nodular regenerative hyperplasia
- Pseudolipoma
- Leiomyoma
- Lymphangioma
- Inflammatory pseudotumor
- Biliary cystadenoma

- does it contain hepatocytes?
- does it contain Kupffer cells?
- is there a central scar?

The characteristics of the more common benign lesions are summarized in Table 9.2.

In uncertain cases, additional information may be obtained from angiography or radionucleotide studies. Lesions that are difficult to classify after radiological evaluation may be further evaluated by biopsy or reassessed radiologically after intervals of 3–6 months. Lesions are considered to be benign if the dimensions and characteristics of the lesion(s) remain constant during that period. It is not uncommon for individuals to have a combination of benign lesions.

Benign liver tumors

Hemangiomas are the most common of all the benign focal lesions and are present in at least 1% of the population. The size is variable but most are solitary, are less than 5 cm in diameter and remain static in size over time. Hemangiomas are most commonly found near the capsule of the right lobe. Classic lesions can be diagnosed with a high

TABLE 9.2

Characteristics of benign liver tumors

Solid	Vascular	Hepatocytes	Kupffer cells	Central scar
Hemangioma				
Complex	Yes	No	No	No
Focal nodular hyperplasia				
Yes	Yes	Yes	Yes	Yes
Adenoma				
Yes	Yes	Yes	No	Maybe
Cyst				
No	No	No	No	No

degree of confidence with any of the radiological techniques, but occasionally complex lesions require extensive investigation. Dynamic scanning using contrast shows a pattern of filling from the edge to the center. The overwhelming majority of hemangiomas do not need either extended surveillance or treatment. Occasionally a hemangioma may become so large that intervention is indicated; embolization and surgery are the treatments most commonly utilized.

Focal nodular hyperplasia is the most frequent of the benign solid liver tumors and is most commonly encountered in women during their reproductive years. There is a weak association with exposure to the oral contraceptive pill. The typical lesion is solitary, measures 3–5 cm in diameter and has a characteristic central scar that may be visualized on scanning. About 15% of patients report vague abdominal pain and the remainder are asymptomatic. Unlike adenomas, there is no risk of rupture or malignant transformation and these lesions do not need specific therapy.

Adenomas are rare – about 300 are diagnosed annually in the USA – but are the most clinically relevant of the benign tumors. The development of adenoma is closely linked to use of the oral contraceptive pill in women and androgen therapy in men. Regression after cessation of exposure to the hormonal stimulus may occur but is not consistent. Unlike focal nodular hyperplasia, these lesions have the potential to grow, hemorrhage and rupture. The latter two complications may present with severe abdominal pain. Pregnancy increases the risk of rupture, so regular ultrasound surveillance is recommended.

Although rare, malignant transformation is a concern and is one of the reasons to consider resection. Surgical resection is recommended if an adenoma exceeds 10 cm in diameter; however, this is not an option when the lesions are multiple and distributed throughout both lobes of the liver, a condition referred to as adenomatosis.

Cysts

Simple cysts are common and are found in 2.5% of the population. They are most likely to be seen in older women and vary in size from

1 to 20 cm. Most are asymptomatic unless very large or complicated by infection or hemorrhage into the cyst. The appearance on ultrasonography is characteristic as a well-defined echo-free lesion with posterior acoustic enhancement. Cysts tend to recur after simple drainage procedures, but may not do so if sclerosant is injected into the cavity. Defenestration or surgical removal are alternative therapies.

Polycystic liver disease may occur in isolation or in association with polycystic kidney disease. Some cases are associated with congenital hepatic fibrosis. The extent of the cystic change is variable but can lead to near total replacement of the liver parenchyma. Liver transplantation has been performed in cases where the sheer bulk of the liver has become problematic and in cases of venous outflow obstruction (Budd–Chiari syndrome; see Chapter 2, Acute liver disease). These cysts can also be complicated by hemorrhage and infection.

Choledochal cysts are congenital cystic dilations of the biliary tree. Pain or jaundice are the most common presenting symptoms, typically in young adults. There may be coexisting congenital hepatic fibrosis. Surgical resection may be required.

Infections and abscesses

Pyogenic liver abscesses are discrete pockets of infection within the substance of the liver tissue. Dissemination from a primary source of infection is the most common underlying cause, and portal pyemia complicating intra-abdominal infection such as appendicitis or diverticulitis accounts for a substantial proportion of cases. There are two patterns of abscess: multiple small abscesses distributed throughout the liver, and larger discrete abscesses, which have a predilection for the right lobe. The latter are readily apparent on scanning the liver, but small abscesses may be difficult to detect.

Drainage of larger abscesses is achieved percutaneously or surgically and is the mainstay of treatment. Despite effective drainage, protracted periods of antibiotic therapy are required to eradicate the infection. Antibiotics are the only effective therapy for the smaller, diffuse pattern of infection. Abscesses that develop as a complication of cholangitis may be in direct communication with the biliary tree, and effective drainage may be achieved by endoscopic measures taken to address the cause of the underlying biliary obstruction.

In liver transplant recipients, liver abscesses are either a manifestation of hepatic artery thrombosis or severe cholangitis. The impairment of perfusion that follows hepatic artery occlusion renders antibiotic therapy ineffective, and retransplantation is usually required.

Amebic abscess is caused by *Entamoeba histolytica* and is most common in tropical and subtropical climates. The initial infection may be associated with a diarrheal illness. Discomfort in the right upper quadrant and fever are the main presenting symptoms. The abscess can usually be detected on ultrasonography and is most frequently found in the right lobe. The diagnosis is confirmed by serology. Most cases respond to therapy with metronidazole or tinidazole; drainage or surgery are reserved for difficult cases.

Hydatid disease is caused by infestation with the tapeworm *Echinococcus granulosus*, which resides in dogs but can infect sheep and humans. Symptoms, usually subtle, include fever and abdominal pain. The cysts are detected on ultrasonography or CT and often have characteristic 'daughter cysts' attached to the wall of the dominant cyst. The diagnosis is suggested by positive serology. Percutaneous aspiration of the cysts is not advised. Initial management is with mebendazole or albendazole but many cases will require surgical resection.

Cholangitis is infection in the biliary tree and is usually associated with an obstruction to bile flow (e.g. stone in the common bile duct, benign stricture or malignant disease). The classical triad of symptoms is:
- fever and rigors
- jaundice
- pain in the right upper quadrant.

The treatment consists of antibiotic therapy and, if possible, relief of the underlying obstruction via endoscopic retrograde cholangiopancreatography. Cholecystectomy is indicated in patients with gallstone disease.

Key points – benign liver tumors, cysts, infections and abscesses

- Benign liver lesions are relatively common.
- Most lesions identified are unrelated to the symptoms under investigation.
- Hemangiomas and focal nodular hyperplasia are managed conservatively.
- Adenomas are closely linked to hormone therapy and require surveillance and occasionally surgical resection.

Key reference

Karani J. Benign tumours and cystic diseases of the liver. In: O'Grady JG, Lake JR, Howdle PD, eds. *Comprehensive Clinical Hepatology*. London: Mosby, 2000:ch 24.1, pp 1–13.

10 Hepatocellular carcinoma

Epidemiology and pathogenesis

Hepatocellular carcinoma (hepatoma, HCC) is a malignancy of hepatocytes. Although relatively uncommon in the USA (incidence of approximately 3 per 100 000), HCC figures prominently in the morbidity and mortality of the developing world – an incidence of approximately 100 per 100 000 in Asia and Africa has been reported, but this figure may be lower than the true incidence because of under-reporting. Marked geographic variation in incidence is largely due to variation in the risk factors that predispose an individual to the tumor (Table 10.1). Most cases of HCC occur in liver that is already cirrhotic. Thus, patients with advanced viral hepatitis, hemochromatosis or alcoholic liver disease are at risk. Hepatitis B presents a unique risk, as there is evidence that a tumor may develop in the absence of cirrhosis – presumably via direct integration of viral DNA into the host genome.

Clinical presentation

HCC is difficult to diagnose until there is widespread involvement of the liver. Symptoms and changes on physical examination are not specific, and are usually attributed to the underlying liver disorder (Table 10.2). The standard liver biochemical markers are not particularly helpful, although sudden elevations in bilirubin or alkaline phosphatase may suggest obstruction of the biliary tree by a tumor. In the absence of

TABLE 10.1

Risk factors for hepatocellular carcinoma

- Cirrhosis of any etiology
- Hepatitis B
- Hepatitis C
- Hemochromatosis
- Aflatoxin exposure

TABLE 10.2

Symptoms and signs of hepatocellular carcinoma

- Abdominal pain
- Hepatomegaly
- Weight loss
- Ascites
- Weakness

- Splenomegaly
- Abdominal swelling
- Wasting
- Jaundice
- Fever

From Kew MC, Hepatic tumors and cysts. In: Feldman M, Friedman LS, Sleisenger MH, eds. *Sleisenger & Fordtran's Gastrointestinal and Liver Disease*, 7th edn. Philadelphia: WB Saunders, 2003:ch 81, p 1578.

specific clinical findings, most hepatologists suspect HCC when there is a change in the expected clinical course of a patient with otherwise stable liver disease. Paraneoplastic syndromes related to HCC may also give clues to the diagnosis (Table 10.3).

Diagnosis

Because of the non-specific clinical presentation, the diagnosis of HCC is typically made using serum tumor markers, imaging studies and, at times, liver biopsy.

TABLE 10.3

Paraneoplastic syndromes related to hepatocellular carcinoma

- Hypoglycemia
- Hypercalcemia
- Erythrocytosis
- Neuroendocrine syndromes (carcinoid, VIPoma)
- Skin changes (Leser–Trelat sign, pityriasis rotunda, etc.)

VIP, vasoactive intestinal polypeptide.

Immature (fetal) liver cells synthesize alpha fetoprotein (AFP). Malignant hepatocytes resemble immature hepatocytes, and AFP is an important marker for HCC. Serum levels of AFP greater than 200 ng/mL are highly suggestive of HCC. Lower levels can be seen with any liver disease that provokes hepatocyte regeneration (ongoing hepatitis, cirrhosis). AFP is also produced during pregnancy and by some germ-cell tumors. Unfortunately, not all HCCs produce AFP; 30–40% of patients with HCC have normal AFP levels, which considerably limits the usefulness of AFP for screening.

Imaging studies are particularly useful when confirming a diagnosis of HCC. Ultrasonography is inexpensive, safe and convenient. Although widely used, its sensitivity is only about 50%. Computed tomography, especially when used with rapid scanning techniques, helps to identify and stage the tumor. It has better sensitivity than ultrasonography, making it particularly useful for detecting small tumors. Magnetic resonance imaging, angiography and positron emission tomography may each provide additional information. Because of rapidly changing imaging technology and variability in local availability, consultation with a radiologist is strongly recommended.

Many hepatologists believe that suspected HCC lesions (suspected on the basis of imaging characteristics, growth patterns and elevated AFP levels) should not be biopsied for fear that the biopsy may spread the tumor. Unfortunately, however, clinicians are usually faced with presentations that are less clear, and needle biopsy of the liver is required to confirm the diagnosis.

Screening

Available data do not support the efficacy of screening for HCC. Nevertheless, because there are few symptoms or objective signs of the tumor before it has progressed to an incurable stage, and because screening is associated with few risks, many practitioners offer screening to their patients. Patients with established cirrhosis, particularly if from viral hepatitis or hemochromatosis, are at the highest risk for HCC. It is therefore reasonable that these candidates be screened, typically with an ultrasound scan and AFP measurement every 6–12 months.

Treatment

If tumors are small and there is no evidence of extrahepatic spread, surgical resection may be considered. Unfortunately, however, few patients with HCC have resectable tumors or sufficient hepatic reserve to tolerate a partial hepatectomy, and approximately 50% of tumors will have recurred at 5 years. Orthotopic liver transplantation may be an option for some patients, provided there is no evidence of extrahepatic spread and the patient is an otherwise good candidate for transplantation (see Chapter 12, Liver transplantation). The prognosis is best for patients with either a single small tumor (less than 5 cm) or no more than three lesions, each smaller than 3 cm.

Many patients with HCC are not candidates for either liver transplantation or surgical resection, and systemic chemotherapy has limited, if any, efficacy. Hormone therapy with tamoxifen and immunotherapy with interferon have shown promising results. Embolizing the tumor (to interrupt its blood supply) or infusing chemotherapeutic agents directly into the tumor via the hepatic artery have been offered by specialized centers, with variable results. Percutaneous ethanol injection is widely used to palliate small tumors. Other direct treatments such as radiofrequency or microwave ablation and cryosurgery have yielded variable results. Therapy for most patients with HCC is best provided by specialized centers, where patients may be considered for inclusion in randomized controlled trials.

Other primary hepatic tumors

Hepatoblastoma is the most common primary hepatic malignancy in children. It usually presents with abdominal swelling, weight loss and failure to thrive, and serum AFP is almost always elevated. Hepatoblastoma is an aggressive tumor and is associated with a poor prognosis; its response to systemic chemotherapy or radiation is inconsistent. If detected in early stages, a well-encapsulated tumor may be surgically resectable. Liver transplantation may be an option for some patients.

Angiosarcoma is an uncommon malignancy of hepatic mesenchymal cells. Histologically, the tumor is characterized by numerous blood-filled cystic structures lined with malignant endothelial cells. Exposure to arsenic (from insecticides or medications), thorium dioxide and vinyl chloride monomer are well-known risk factors. Like hepatoblastomas, angiosarcomas grow rapidly and are rarely discovered while resectable. Chemotherapy and radiation are usually not helpful, and the prognosis is poor.

Key points – hepatocellular carcinoma

- Hepatocellular carcinoma is a worrisome complication of advanced liver disease.
- Hepatocellular carcinoma often has few specific symptoms or signs.
- Hepatocellular carcinoma should be suspected in patients with an unexpected worsening of liver disease.
- Screening for hepatocellular carcinoma is of unclear utility, but is widely practiced. Regular checking of serum alpha fetoprotein levels and hepatic ultrasound scanning are acceptable.
- Curative treatment by resection or transplantation is an option, but not always possible.

Key references

Bailey MA, Brunt EM. Hepatocellular carcinoma: predisposing conditions and precursor lesions. *Gastroenterol Clin N Am* 2002;31:641–64.

Di Bisceglie AM. Hepatitis C and hepatocellular carcinoma. *Hepatology* 1997;26(3 suppl 1): 34–8S.

Okuda K. Hepatocellular carcinoma. *J Hepatol* 200;32(suppl 1):225–37.

Sherman M. Surveillance for hepatocellular carcinoma. *Semin Oncol* 2001;28:450–9.

Wall WJ. Liver transplantation for hepatic and biliary malignancy. *Semin Liver Dis* 2000;20:425–36.

The interaction between pregnancy and the liver has a number of aspects:

- physiological changes
- pregnancy-related liver dysfunction (Figure 11.1)
- management of established chronic liver disease during pregnancy
- coincidental acute liver disease.

Physiological changes

Pregnancy produces cutaneous signs associated with chronic liver disease, including palmar erythema and spider nevi. The majority of the laboratory parameters of liver function remain normal, but:

- alkaline phosphatase increases from the seventh month to term
- serum albumin decreases by up to 20%.

Pregnancy-related liver dysfunction

Hyperemesis gravidarum. Severe vomiting in the first trimester of pregnancy may be associated with abnormal liver function tests,

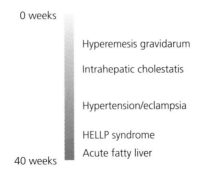

Figure 11.1 Schematic representation of most likely time for development of pregnancy-related liver dysfunction. HELLP, hemolysis, elevated liver enzymes, low platelet count.

typically a modest elevation in the serum aminotransferases (up to 5 times the upper limit of normal) and possibly an increased serum bilirubin. The abnormalities resolve with rehydration and control of the vomiting, and no specific therapy is required for the liver.

Cholestasis of pregnancy complicates up to 1% of pregnancies and accounts for 20% of cases of jaundice during pregnancy. It typically presents with itch in the second and third trimesters. Jaundice subsequently develops in association with pale stools and dark urine. The liver function profile shows a marked increase in serum alkaline phosphatase and possibly hyperbilirubinemia. A vitamin-K-responsive coagulopathy may be a manifestation of decreased absorption of fat-soluble vitamins. Management involves control of the pruritus with colestyramine or ursodeoxycholic acid. Cholestasis is likely to recur in subsequent pregnancies and with subsequent use of the oral contraceptive pill.

Acute fatty liver of pregnancy presents in the third trimester and is most common in first pregnancies and with a male fetus. The incidence is also increased with twin pregnancies. The presenting symptoms include vomiting, abdominal pain and evidence of fluid retention. Severe cases develop features of acute liver failure (jaundice, hypoglycemia, encephalopathy) in association with evidence of disseminated intravascular coagulation syndrome and renal failure.

Acute fatty liver is a mitochondrial cytopathy; the pathogenesis has recently been linked to a genetic deficiency of long-chain 3-hydroxyacyl coenzyme-A dehydrogenase. The liver function profile shows increased serum bilirubin in association with a mild-to-moderate increase in serum aminotransferases. The uric acid level is characteristically elevated. The fatty infiltration of the liver may be apparent on ultrasonography or computed tomography of the liver. Biopsy is rarely required to establish the diagnosis.

Termination of the pregnancy is central to successful management of the condition – clinical improvement is usually apparent within 24 hours of delivery. Severe cases require intravenous fluids, antibiotics and supportive measures for liver and renal insufficiency. The prognosis is good, even in severe cases, and rescue with emergency liver transplantation is needed only occasionally.

Hypertension and eclampsia. Hypertension is a key element of pre-eclampsia and eclampsia, with additional features including proteinuria, edema and seizures. The frequency and severity of liver dysfunction increase with the severity of the syndrome. The dominant abnormality is in the serum aminotransferases, which may be very high and in the range associated with acute hepatitis.

The mechanism of injury is fibrinoid necrosis; in severe cases, focal areas of ischemia are identified on biopsy and radiological assessment. Acute liver failure, hepatic infarction and rupture are all recognized complications. Renal failure and thrombocytopenia are other common features of severe disease. Management involves control of the hypertension and early termination of the pregnancy. Emergency liver transplantation may be indicated.

HELLP syndrome is so named for:
- hemolysis
- elevated liver enzymes
- low platelet count.

There is considerable overlap between this syndrome and hypertension-related liver dysfunction, and management is effectively the same as for the latter condition (see above).

Pre-existing liver disease

Amenorrhea and infertility are common in patients with cirrhosis. Conception tends to be a testimony to the degree of preservation of liver function. Intuitively, one would consider bleeding from varices to be a significant risk, given the expansion of the intravascular volume and increasing intra-abdominal pressure. However, this has not been clearly demonstrated to be the case, and even the stresses of vaginal delivery are not associated with an increased risk of hemorrhage. The individual risk of bleeding should be assessed endoscopically for each woman, and appropriate prophylactic measures instituted. In most cases, this will mean consideration of propranolol therapy, but occasionally individuals with mucosal stigmata associated with a high-risk status may require endoscopic intervention and obliteration of varices.

Autoimmune hepatitis tends to be fairly quiescent during pregnancy, with flares in disease activity observed in fewer than 10% of cases. However, primary biliary cirrhosis may deteriorate during pregnancy.

Coincidental acute liver disease

- **Acute viral hepatitis.** The clinical courses of hepatitis A and B are unaltered by pregnancy, but mortality is increased with hepatitis E.
- **Budd–Chiari syndrome.** Pregnancy and the postpartum period are times of increased risk for the development of hepatic vein thrombosis in susceptible individuals.
- **Gallstones.** Pregnancy facilitates the development of gallstones, which are found in up to 10% of pregnant women. Biliary obstruction should be managed endoscopically rather than surgically during the pregnancy.
- **Acute liver failure,** unrelated to the pregnancy, may develop after deliberate or accidental acetaminophen (paracetamol) overdose, infection with hepatitis E or other coincidental reasons. Fetal mortality is very high. Maternal care is standard for the condition, and successful liver transplants during pregnancy have been reported.
- **Adenoma.** Surveillance during pregnancy is recommended because of the associated stimulus to growth.

Key points – pregnancy and the liver

- Three classical syndromes of liver dysfunction are associated with late pregnancy: acute fatty liver, hypertension/eclampsia-related dysfunction and HELLP syndrome, but considerable overlap exists between them.
- Cholestasis of pregnancy is a recurrent disorder which is associated with increased fetal mortality.
- Pregnancy is surprisingly well tolerated by women with chronic liver disease.

Key reference

Su GL, Van Dyke R. Liver disease and pregnancy. In: *Liver Disease: Diagnosis and Management.* Bacon BR, Di Bisceglie AM, eds. Philadelphia: Churchill Livingstone, 2000:344–51.

Almost 5000 liver transplants are performed each year in the USA. After transplant, most patients enjoy long-term survival and dramatic improvements in quality of life. Many patients with advanced liver disease, however, are not candidates for liver transplantation, and there remains a serious shortage of donor organs.

Referring physicians should understand the importance of timing for liver transplantation, be familiar with its indications and contraindications and be comfortable with a pretransplantation evaluation.

Indications and contraindications

Liver transplantation may be a viable option for patients with advanced liver disease of almost any etiology. In the USA, the most common indications for transplantation resulting from chronic liver disease are viral hepatitis and alcoholic liver disease (ALD) (Table 12.1). Advanced liver disease that has resulted from acute disorders may also require liver transplantation (Table 12.2).

TABLE 12.1

Indications for liver transplantation: chronic conditions

Advanced liver disease due to:	Metabolic liver diseases:
• Chronic viral hepatitis	• Wilson's disease
• Alcoholic liver disease	• Hemochromatosis
• Autoimmune hepatitis	• α_1 antitrypsin deficiency
• Primary biliary cirrhosis	• Familial hypercholesterolemia
• Primary sclerosing cholangitis	
• Hepatocellular carcinoma	

TABLE 12.2

Indications for liver transplantation: acute conditions/fulminant hepatic failure

- Viral hepatitis A, B, C, etc.
- Drug-induced liver disease
- Toxin-induced liver disease
- Wilson's disease
- Acute fatty liver of pregnancy
- Reye's syndrome

TABLE 12.3

Contraindications for liver transplant

Absolute

- Active substance/alcohol abuse
- Extrahepatic malignancy
- Ongoing sepsis
- Advanced cardiac or pulmonary disease
- Psychosocial or social difficulties that would interfere with compliance

Relative

- Advanced age
- Severe obesity
- Poor functional status
- Human immunodeficiency virus infection

It is important to select candidates who can tolerate the significant physiological, emotional and social stressors that often accompany liver transplantation. Accepted contraindications are listed in Table 12.3. An extensive pretransplant evaluation is required to assess the patient's physiological, social and psychiatric reserves, as liver transplantation will place significant stress on these factors (Table 12.4).

Timing of liver transplantation

Referral criteria for acute and chronic liver disease differ. Acute, severe liver disease (fulminant liver failure) is defined as the rapid development of jaundice and encephalopathy in a patient with no history of liver disease. Acute viral hepatitis and drug-induced liver injury are common causes. Criteria have been developed to aid clinician referral of patients with fulminant hepatic failure (Table 12.5). In general, patients with acute liver disease complicated by encephalopathy should be transferred to a liver transplant center for continued observation and preparation for transplant if needed.

With regard to chronic liver disease, it is best to select patients for liver transplant whose survival would otherwise be dramatically limited. It must be noted, however, that advanced liver disease itself causes systemic changes that may limit the success of liver transplantation. Thus, the clinician must select patients who are most in need of liver transplant, *and* are likely to survive the procedure. The Child's score (Table 12.6) predicts survival for patients with advanced cirrhosis. Patients with a score greater than 7 are likely to benefit from consultation at a liver transplant center. The model for end-stage liver

---

TABLE 12.4

Pretransplant evaluation

- Routine evaluation of hepatic, renal, thyroid and hematologic function
- Serology for human immunodeficiency virus, hepatitis B and C viruses and cytomegalovirus
- Chest radiograph, pulmonary function tests
- Electrocardiogram, echocardiogram and possibly stress test
- Doppler ultrasound evaluation of liver blood vessels
- Contrast computed tomography of abdomen
- Psychosocial and substance abuse evaluation

TABLE 12.5

Indications for liver transplant: acute liver disease

Acetaminophen (paracetamol) overdose

- pH < 7.3 (irrespective of grade of encephalopathy) OR
- PT > 100 seconds and serum creatinine > 300 μmol/L (3.4 mg/dL) in patients with grade III or IV encephalopathy

Other patients

- PT > 100 seconds (irrespective of grade of encephalopathy) OR
- Any three of the following variables (irrespective of grade of encephalopathy):
  - age < 10 or > 40 years
  - etiology: non-A, non-B hepatitis, halothane hepatitis, idiosyncratic drug reactions
  - duration of jaundice before onset of encephalopathy > 7days
  - PT > 50 seconds
  - serum bilirubin concentration > 300 μmol/L (17.6 mg/dL)

PT, prothrombin time.
From O'Grady et al. 1989.

disease (MELD score) predicts survival of patients with cirrhosis using serum bilirubin and creatinine levels and the international normalized ratio (INR). (Calculators are available on the internet, for example at www.unos.org/resources/meldpeldcalculator.asp.) Most centers now use the MELD score to prioritize patients awaiting liver transplant. A similar score for pediatric end-stage liver disease (PELD score) has also been developed.

Other criteria, including the development of frequent portal hypertensive bleeding, spontaneous bacterial peritonitis or intractable ascites, should prompt referral for liver transplantation. Intractable pruritis, fatigue and bone disease associated with cholestasis may also identify potential candidates.

TABLE 12.6

Determination of Child's score, used to predict the survival of patients with severe cirrhosis

Clinical finding	Points		
	1	2	3
Encephalopathy	None	Grade 1–2	Grade 3–4
Ascites	None	Mild	Moderate
Bilirubin (mg/dL)	< 2	2–3	> 3
(μmol/L)	< 34	34–51	> 51
Albumin (mg/dL)	> 3.5	2.8–3.5	< 2.8
PT (seconds prolonged)	1–3	4–6	> 6

Values in the columns are added for the clinical findings listed.

- Child's class A   5 or 6 points   Patient has well-maintained liver function and excellent expected survival
- Child's class B   7, 8 or 9 points   Reduced survival
- Child's class C   10+ points   Very poor prognosis

Special concerns

Viral hepatitis. Patients with hepatitis B and C make up a significant proportion of those undergoing orthotopic liver transplantation. As expected, these viruses usually reappear in the transplanted organ. Hepatitis B is particularly aggressive, and its recurrence may result in early graft failure or death. Its suppression with hepatitis B immuno-globulin or antiretroviral agents such as lamivudine and adefovir offers new hope to patients previously excluded from transplantation.

Hepatitis C is an extraordinarily common virus that may be responsible for, or complicate (in the case of ALD or following transfusion), a patient's liver disease. Although reinfection of the graft is nearly universal, outcomes for these patients are much better than for those with hepatitis B. Hepatitis C always recurs after transplantation with variable consequences, but some patients develop accelerated disease such that graft survival rates are inferior to those for other etiologies 8 years after transplantation. Nevertheless, hepatitis C is not a contraindication to liver transplantation.

Alcoholism. Transplantation for patients with ALD remains controversial. Many clinicians feel that the social and psychological stresses associated with liver transplant would lead to recidivism. These concerns are unconfirmed, however, and it appears that fewer than 20% of well-selected patients return to problem drinking. Survival of patients with ALD following transplantation appears to be comparable to that of transplant patients with non-alcoholic liver disease. Most transplant centers require at least 6 months' abstinence before consideration for liver transplantation.

Living donor liver transplant (LDLT). The lack of available transplant organs often prevents liver transplantation for approved candidates. Alternatively, an LDLT may be considered. This allows an elective operation and access to more organs and grafts in excellent condition. In LDLT, the right lobe of the donor's (usually a close relative) liver is excised and transplanted into the recipient. Because of the liver's rapid regenerative capacity, both organs regenerate to a size appropriate for metabolic activity. LDLT is a technically demanding procedure, performed at a few specialized centers. Unfortunately, donor morbidity and mortality, although unlikely, are possible.

Long-term management of liver transplant recipients

The number of liver transplants being performed annually worldwide is around 10 000. It is becoming increasingly likely that medical practitioners will encounter liver transplant recipients on an occasional basis and will need some insight into aspects that differentiate these individuals from their normal patient population. Issues relating to graft function, as well as other complex medical matters, are managed by the transplant centers. However, the recognition and early management of some of these problems will remain in the hands of primary care physicians and non-specialist staff.

Immunosuppression. The need for long-term immunosuppression is one of the main features of these patients. Liver transplant recipients tend to be less aggressively immunosuppressed than recipients of other solid organ transplants. Nevertheless, there are issues with:

- immunosuppression per se
- effects of individual immunosuppressive drugs.

Long-term immunosuppression increases the risk of opportunistic infections and malignant disease (Table 12.7). Where indicated, the interval between screenings for malignancy should be reduced (e.g. cervical smears, or colonoscopy in patients with ulcerative colitis, every year rather than every 3 years). Opportunistic infections are relatively uncommon, and the presenting signs are often non-specific. However, it is clear that early recognition is important so that effective therapy can be commenced. This perspective on opportunistic infections is presented on the basis of the possible presenting clinical problems.

Cough and other respiratory symptoms are a common presentation; most cases are caused by familiar community infections. Vaccination against influenza is recommended for liver transplant recipients and should reduce the incidence of influenza in these patients. Antibiotic therapy is widely used to prevent or treat superimposed bacterial bronchitis, which is a common sequel to viral respiratory tract infections. Opportunistic infections should be considered if:

- symptoms do not resolve within the expected time period

TABLE 12.7

Malignant diseases that are more common in liver transplant recipients

- Post-transplant lymphoproliferative disease or lymphoma
- Skin malignancies
- Oropharyngeal carcinoma (especially in alcohol consumers)
- Colonic carcinoma in patients with ulcerative colitis
- Risk-factor-associated malignancy (e.g. lung cancer in smokers)

- shortness of breath develops, particularly if this is disproportionate to findings on chest radiograph
- associated findings occur (e.g. lymphadenopathy).

Cytomegalovirus, *Pneumocystis carinii*, aspergillosis and mycobacterial infections are the main opportunistic infections that present with respiratory symptoms.

- Infection with cytomegalovirus tends to occur within the first year of transplantation and is typically associated with a very high fever.
- *Pneumocystis carinii* presents with a dry cough and shortness of breath.
- Mycobacterial infections may present with hemoptysis or have associated lymphadenopathy.

Diarrhea is another frequent problem and is usually explained by drug toxicity or common infections. The latter are generally well tolerated, and management is as standard for immunocompetent individuals. However, diarrhea may also be the presentation of an opportunistic infection. *Clostridium difficile* is common in the early post-transplant period when exposure to broad-spectrum antibiotics is high. Reactivation of the infection can occur in the community, and a stool sample should be screened in patients known to have had previous infection. Cytomegalovirus can cause gastroenteritis, and this should be considered in patients with high fevers, abdominal pain or rectal bleeding.

Lymphadenopathy. Lymphoma or post-transplant lympho-proliferative disease (PTLD) must be considered in any patient with unexplained lymphadenopathy. This is the most common malignant disease after liver transplantation and can present at any time. The risk of developing PTLD correlates roughly with the cumulative intensity of immunosuppression, but all patients should be considered at risk. Suspected cases should be referred immediately to specialist centers. Mycobacterial infections, both typical and atypical, should be considered if there are associated respiratory symptoms and when the distribution is predominantly in the cervical region.

Pyrexia of unknown origin. Unexplained fevers, especially in association with non-specific systemic symptoms such as anorexia and weight loss, may be indicative of PTLD.

Immunosuppressive drugs. The majority of liver transplant recipients are maintained on an immunosuppression regimen based on calcineurin inhibition with either tacrolimus or ciclosporin. These may be used in combination with other drugs to increase potency or, more commonly, to reduce the toxicity of individual drugs. Agents for maintenance immunosuppression include prednisone, azathioprine and the newer agents mycophenolate and sirolimus. Transplant centers are usually responsible for monitoring drug dosing.

Side effects. All of the immunosuppressive drugs have potential side effects (Table 12.8). However, some of these are sufficiently common in the context of liver transplantation (e.g. headache and diarrhea) that extensive investigation is unnecessary. Other potential side effects require careful prospective monitoring, with adjustments to the immunosuppressive regimen if necessary. A typical example is the nephrotoxicity associated with long-term use of calcineurin inhibitors – up to 25% of liver transplant recipients have chronic renal failure 10 years after transplantation. This is being addressed by reducing reliance on calcineurin inhibitors.

TABLE 12.8

Side effects of long-term immunosuppressive regimens

General
- Malignant disease
- Opportunistic infections

Common and possibly considered tolerable
- Tremor
- Headache
- Diarrhea
- Hirsutism
- Gingival hyperplasia
- Alopecia

Common but requiring intervention
- Hypertension
- Diabetes mellitus
- Gout
- Weight gain/obesity

Requiring specific monitoring
- Impaired renal function
- Hyperlipidemia
- Osteoporosis

Drug interactions. The potential for drug interactions is great, but in patients taking ciclosporin or tacrolimus the following two points are of particular importance.

• Avoid non-steroidal anti-inflammatory drugs and any antibiotic ending in '-mycin' (e.g. clarithromycin) because of the threat of renal failure (even with short-term use).

• Among herbal remedies, St John's wort should be avoided.

Disease recurrence. Many liver diseases have the potential to recur after liver transplantation (Table 12.9). The liver transplant center will normally screen for recurrent disease, but some diseases may first become apparent to the primary care physician (e.g. ALD), whereas others may be comanaged in the community (e.g. hepatitis C).

Vaccinations. Only live or attenuated vaccines are contraindicated.

Contraception and reproduction. Sexual function in men and fertility in premenopausal women is usually restored after liver transplantation. Intra-uterine contraceptive devices may cause infection and should be used with care. Hormonal contraception is

---

TABLE 12.9

Diseases that commonly recur after liver transplantation

Common, may threaten graft/patient survival

• Hepatitis C (near-universal, variable progression)
• Hepatitis B (15% despite prophylaxis)
• Excessive alcohol consumption (15%)
• Hepatocellular carcinoma (15–20%)
• Other malignant diseases

Lower impact on graft function

• Alcohol consumption
• Autoimmune hepatitis
• Primary biliary cirrhosis
• Primary sclerosing cholangitis
• Budd–Chiari syndrome

contraindicated in patients with prothrombotic disorders, particularly Budd–Chiari syndrome. Pregnancy is generally well tolerated but transplant patients have a higher incidence of some complications (e.g. hypertension, low birth weight).

Dietary restrictions pertinent to chronic liver disease (e.g. salt or protein restriction) no longer apply. Restriction of calorie intake is important in the 20–25% of patients with accelerated weight gain or obesity. Dietary adjustments are needed in patients with diabetes mellitus, hyperlipidemia or hypertension. Some foods are contraindicated because of the risk of infection (e.g. paté, uncooked shellfish, unpasteurized cheeses).

Key points – liver transplantation

- Liver transplantation is effective for a wide range of liver diseases.
- Hepatitis B and C do not contraindicate transplantation.
- Thorough assessment is mandatory, and must cover physiological, social and psychiatric comorbidity.
- Many diseases recur after transplantation, but with variable consequences.
- Careful attention to the complications of immunosuppression is of great importance; as well as possible opportunistic infections, drug interactions and side effects can occur.
- Limitations to lifestyle after transplantation are remarkably few.

Key references

Abecassis M, Adams M, Adams P et al. Consensus statement on the liver organ donor. *JAMA* 2000;284:2919–26.

Luxon BA. Liver transplantation. Who should be referred – and when? *Postgrad Med* 1997;102:103–13.

Neuberger J, Schulz KH, Day C et al. Transplantation for alcoholic liver disease. *J Hepatol* 2002;36:130-7.

O'Grady JG, Alexander GJ, Hayllar KM, Williams R. Early indicators of prognosis in fulminant hepatic failure. *Gastroenterology* 1989:97;439–45.

Prince MI, Hudson M. Liver transplantation for chronic liver disease: advances and controversies in an era of organ shortages. *Postgrad Med J* 2002;78:135–41.

Rosen HR, Shackleton CR, Martin P. Indications for and timing of liver transplantation. *Med Clin North Am* 1996;80:1069–102.

Useful resources

American Association for the
Study of Liver Diseases
1729 King Street, Suite 200
Alexandria, VA 22314, USA
Tel: +1 703 288 9766
Fax: +1 703 299 9622
aasld@easld.org
www.aasld.org

American Gastroenterological
Association
7910 Woodmont Avenue, 7th floor
Bethesda, MD 20814, USA
Tel: +1 301 654 2055
Fax: +1 301 652 3890
www.gastro.org

American Liver Foundation
75 Maiden Lane, Suite 203
New York, NY 10038, USA
Tel: +1 212 668 1000
Fax: +1 212 483 8179
www.liverfoundation.org

British Association for the Study
of the Liver and
British Liver Nurses Forum
2 Southampton Road
Ringwood BH24 1HY, UK
Tel: +44 (0)870 7708028
Fax: +44 (0)1425 481335
www.basl.org.uk

British Liver Trust
info@britishlivertrust.org.uk
www.britishlivertrust.org.uk

British Society of
Gastroenterology
3 St Andrew's Place
Regent's Park
London NW1 4LB, UK
Tel: +44 (0)20 7387 3534
Fax: +44 (0)20 7487 3734
www.bsg.org.uk

Cancerbackup
3 Bath Place
Rivington Street
London EC2A 3JR, UK
Freephone helpline: 0808 800 1234
Helpline: +44 (0)20 7739 2280
Tel (office): +44 (0)20 7696 9003
Fax: +44 (0)20 7696 9002
www.cancerbackup.org.uk/
cancertype/liver/primarylivercancer

Cancer Help UK
Cancer Information Department
Cancer Research UK
PO Box 123, Lincoln's Inn Fields
London WC2A 3PX, UK
cancer.info@cancer.org.uk
www.cancerhelp.org.uk/help/
default.asp?page=4891

European Association for the Study of the Liver

EASL Liaison Bureau

c/o Kenes International

17 rue du Cendrier, PO Box 1726

CH-1211 Geneva, Switzerland

Tel: +41 (0)22 906 91 51

Fax: +41 (0)22 732 28 52

info@easl.ch

www.easl.ch

European Liver Patients Associations

Rue Royale 296

B-1210 Brussels, Belgium

contact@elpa-info.org

www.elpa-info.org

King's College Hospital Liver Transplant Programme

(information suitable for physicians)

www.kingsch.nhs.uk/livertransplant/index.html

MELD/PELD calculator

www.unos.org/resources/meldpeldcalculator.asp

National Cancer Institute (USA)

www.cancer.gov

National Digestive Diseases Information Clearinghouse (USA)

www.digestive.niddk.nih.gov/ddiseases/a-z.asp

Index

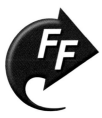

Imagine if every time you wanted to know something you knew where to look...

Over one million copies sold

- Written by world experts
- Concise and practical
- Up to date
- Designed for ease of reading and reference
- Copiously illustrated with useful photographs, diagrams and charts.

Our aim is to make *Fast Facts* the world's most respected medical handbook series. Feedback on how to make titles even more useful is always welcome (feedback@fastfacts.com).

More than 70 *Fast Facts* titles, including:

Asthma
Benign Gynecological Disease (second edition)
Benign Prostatic Hyperplasia (fifth edition)
Bipolar Disorder
Bladder Cancer (second edition)
Bleeding Disorders
Breast Cancer (third edition)
Chronic Obstructive Pulmonary Disease
Colorectal Cancer (second edition)
Contraception (second edition)
Dementia
Depression (second edition)
Diseases of the Pancreas and Biliary Tract
Dyspepsia (second edition)
Eczema and Contact Dermatitis
Endometriosis (second edition)
Epilepsy (third edition)
Erectile Dysfunction (third edition)
Gynecological Oncology
Headaches (second edition)
Hyperlipidemia (third edition)

Hypertension (third edition)
Inflammatory Bowel Disease (second edition)
Irritable Bowel Syndrome (second edition)
Menopause (second edition)
Minor Surgery
Multiple Sclerosis (second edition)
Osteoporosis (fourth edition)
Parkinson's Disease
Prostate Cancer (fourth edition)
Psoriasis (second edition)
Renal Disorders
Respiratory Tract Infection (second edition)
Rheumatoid Arthritis
Schizophrenia (second edition)
Sexual Dysfunction
Sexually Transmitted Infections
Skin Cancer
Smoking Cessation
Soft Tissue Rheumatology
Thyroid Disorders
Urinary Stones

Orders

To order via the website, or to find regional distributors, please go to **www.fastfacts.com**

For telephone orders, please call +44 (0)1752 202301 (Europe), 1 800 247 6553 (USA, toll free) or +1 419 281 1802 (Americas)

Fast Facts

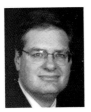

Thomas Mahl MD
University at Buffalo School of Medicine
Buffalo, New York, USA

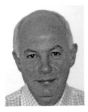

John O'Grady MD
Institute of Liver Studies
King's College School of Medicine
London, UK

Declaration of Independence
This book is as balanced and as practical as we can make it. Ideas
for improvement are always welcome: feedback@fastfacts.com

HEALTH PRESS

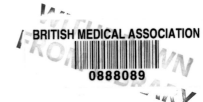

Fast Facts: Liver Disorders
First published May 2006

Text © 2006 Thomas Mahl, John O'Grady
© 2006 in this edition Health Press Limited
Health Press Limited, Elizabeth House, Queen Street, Abingdon,
Oxford OX14 3LN, UK
Tel: +44 (0)1235 523233
Fax: +44 (0)1235 523238

Book orders can be placed by telephone or via the website.
For regional distributors or to order via the website, please go to:
www.fastfacts.com
For telephone orders, please call 01752 202301 (UK), +44 1752 202301 (Europe),
800 247 6553 (USA, toll free) or 419 281 1802 (Canada).

Fast Facts is a trademark of Health Press Limited.

A CIP record for this title is available from the British Library.

ISBN 1-903734-73-8 (978-1-903734-73-5)

Mahl T (Thomas)
Fast Facts: Liver Disorders/
Thomas Mahl, John O'Grady

Medical illustrations by Dee McLean, London, UK.
Typesetting and page layout by Zed, Oxford, UK.
Indexed by Laurence Errington, Edinburgh, UK.
Printed by LinneyPrint Ltd, Mansfield, UK.

Printed with vegetable inks on fully biodegradable and
recyclable paper manufactured from sustainable forests.

444   001
Low emissions
during production

Low   Sustainable
chlorine   forests